The Cleveland Clinic Manual of Dynamic Endocrine Testing

Ahmet Bahadir Ergin • A. Laurence Kennedy
Manjula K. Gupta • Amir H. Hamrahian

The Cleveland Clinic Manual of Dynamic Endocrine Testing

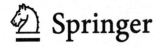 Springer

Ahmet Bahadir Ergin
Department of Endocrinology, Diabetes
and Metabolism
Cleveland Clinic
Cleveland, Ohio
USA

Manjula K. Gupta
Department of Clinical Pathology
Cleveland Clinic
Cleveland, Ohio
USA

A. Laurence Kennedy
Department of Endocrinology, Diabetes
and Metabolism
Cleveland Clinic
Cleveland, Ohio
USA

Amir H. Hamrahian
Department of Endocrinology, Diabetes
and Metabolism
Cleveland Clinic
Cleveland, Ohio
USA

ISBN 978-3-319-13047-7   ISBN 978-3-319-13048-4 (eBook)
DOI 10.1007/978-3-319-13048-4

Library of Congress Control Number: 2014958458

Springer Cham Heidelberg New York Dordrecht London
© Springer International Publishing Switzerland 2015

Printed on acid-free paper

Springer is part of Springer Science+Business Media (www.springer.com)

Preface

Dynamic endocrine testing is the cornerstone of practice in endocrinology and plays an important role in clinical decision-making. Structured and standardized testing protocols are also very important for billing and compliance with high quality standards. However, evidence-based national guidelines for these tests are unfortunately missing.

We in the Cleveland Clinic Department of Endocrinology recently updated our endocrine dynamic testing protocols utilizing current best evidence. These dynamic endocrine tests have been created via a peer review process that included 25 experienced endocrinologists, with each test being discussed at weekly grand rounds. We decided to publish our experience as *The Cleveland Clinic Manual of Dynamic Endocrine Testing*, which will provide an up-to-date practical guide for endocrinologists, nurses, and their staff, both within the USA and outside, who need to perform and interpret dynamic endocrine testing in their everyday practice, as well as medical students, residents, and fellows who have interest in endocrinology.

Each chapter presents of a particular test. Most chapters follow a fairly consistent format covering indication, preparation, materials, interpretation, and caveats. The portion that outlines the actual procedure of the test is presented separately at the end of each chapter for ease of use and reproducibility.

We give special thanks to the physicians and nurses in the Cleveland Clinic Department of Endocrinology, who have contributed to the creation of this valuable book.

Ahmet Bahadir Ergin, MD, CCD, ECNU
A. Laurence Kennedy, MD, FRCP
Manjula K. Gupta, PhD
Amir H. Hamrahian, MD

Contents

Part I
Dynamic Tests in Pituitary/Adrenal Disorders

Chapter 1
ACTH Stimulation Test for Adrenal Insufficiency with Total Cortisol Levels

Indication:	This test is performed to determine whether the adrenal glands can respond normally to ACTH by producing cortisol.
Preparation:	Patients should be off glucocorticoids that potentially interfere with the cortisol assay (hydrocortisone, prednisone) for 24 h pretesting. Dexamethasone may be used.
Materials Needed:	Three (3) gold top tubes labeled as baseline, 30, and/or 60 min

Cortisol: Gold top tube	Cortrosyn 250 mcg Syringes/needles

Assay for Cortisol:	Chemiluminescence immunoassay (CLIA).
Precautions:	Cosyntropin is category C for pregnancy.
Interpretation:	Normal response: Peak stimulated cortisol value > 18 mcg/dl at 30 min [1, 2]. Most patients achieve higher cortisol levels at 60 min compared to 30 min value following 250 mcg cortrosyn administration [2]. Accordingly, a cut-off value of 18 mcg/dL at 60 min may be associated with an increased false positive result.

Caveats:

- Taking oral estrogen may result in elevation of the total cortisol level due to increased corticosteroid binding globulin [3].
- Patients with albumin < 2.5 gr/dL may have a low cortisol level [4].
- Sensitivity for the test is limited in secondary adrenal insufficiency. Specificity is > 95 %, thus a positive cosyntropin test result substantially increases the likelihood that the patient has secondary adrenal insufficiency [5].

© Springer International Publishing Switzerland 2015
A. B. Ergin et al., *The Cleveland Clinic Manual of Dynamic Endocrine Testing,*
DOI 10.1007/978-3-319-13048-4_1

Procedure: Completed as outpatient

1. Draw blood sample for baseline serum cortisol.

2. Give Cortrosyn 250 mcg IM.

3. At 30 and/or 60 min, draw blood samples for serum cortisol.

Physician name and signature: _____

RN performing the procedure: _____

Additional orders by physician: _____

	Baseline	30 min	60 min
Cortisol			

References

1. Grinspoon SK, Biller BM. Clinical review 62: laboratory assessment of adrenal insufficiency. J Clini Endocrinol Metab. 1994;79(4):923–31.
2. May ME, Carey RM. Rapid adrenocorticotropic hormone test in practice. Retrospective review. Am J Med. 1985;79(6):679–84.
3. Klose M, Lange M, Rasmussen AK, et al. Factors influencing the adrenocorticotropin test: Role of contemporary cortisol assays, body composition, and oral contraceptive agents. J Clini Endocrinol Metab. 2007;92(4):1326–33.
4. Hamrahian AH, Oseni TS, Arafah BM. Measurements of serum free cortisol in critically ill patients. N Engl J Med. 2004;350(16):1629–38.
5. Dorin RI, Qualls CR, Crapo LM. Diagnosis of adrenal insufficiency. Ann Intern Med. 2003;139(3):194–204.

Chapter 2
ACTH Stimulation Test for Adrenal Insufficiency with Free Cortisol Levels

Indication:	This test is performed to determine whether the adrenal glands can respond normally to ACTH by producing free cortisol [1, 2]. This test is particularly helpful in patient with albumin <2.5 mg/dL or low CBG.
Preparation:	Patients should be off glucocorticoids that potentially interfere with the cortisol assay (hydrocortisone, prednisone) for 24 h pretesting. Dexamethasone may be used.
Materials Needed:	Three (3) gold top tubes labeled as baseline, 30, and/or 60 min

> **Free cortisol** 0.6 ml:
> Gold top tube.
> Transport: Frozen.
> Remove serum from cells and freeze within 2 hours after collection.

Cortrosyn 250 mcg

Syringes/needles

Assay for Cortisol:	Electrochemiluminescence immunoassay (ECLIA).
Precautions:	Cosyntropin is category C for pregnancy.
Interpretation:	Normal response: Peak stimulated cortisol value >1.2 mcg/dl [3, 4] at 30 or 60 min. Most subjects achieve higher cortisol levels at 60 min compared to the 30 min value following 250 mcg of cosyntropin administration.

© Springer International Publishing Switzerland 2015
A. B. Ergin et al., *The Cleveland Clinic Manual of Dynamic Endocrine Testing*,
DOI 10.1007/978-3-319-13048-4_2

Caveats:

- This cut-off value may not apply to ICU patients. Further studies are needed to establish appropriate levels in such patients. Benefit from glucocorticoid therapy may be beyond adrenal function status in patients with septic shock [1]
- Free cortisol index (FCI) may be used as an alternative to this dynamic test, if free cortisol assay is not available.
- FCI: Total cortisol (nmol/L)/CBG (mg/dl) < 12 suggests adrenal insufficiency [5]. Total cortisol should be measured in the morning between 8–10 am.

Procedure: Completed as outpatient

1. Draw blood sample for baseline serum free cortisol.

2. Give Cortrosyn 250 mcg IM.

3. At 30 and/or 60 min, draw blood samples for serum cortisol.

Physician name and signature: _____

RN performing the procedure: _____

Additional orders by physician: _____

	Baseline	30 min	60 min
Free cortisol			

References

1. Hamrahian AH, Oseni TS, Arafah BM. Measurements of serum free cortisol in critically ill patients. N Engl J Med. 2004;350(16):1629–38.
2. Tan T, Chang L, Woodward A, McWhinney B, Galligan J, Macdonald GA, et al. Characterizing adrenal function using directly measured plasma free cortisol in stable severe liver disease. J Hepatol. 2010;53(5):841–8.
3. Lewis JG, Bagley CJ, Elder PA, Bachmann AW, Torpy DJ. Plasma-free cortisol fraction reflects levels of functioning corticosteroid-binding globulin. Clinica Chimica Acta. 2005;359 (1–2):189–94.
4. Vogeser M, Briegel J, Zachoval R. Dialyzable free cortisol after stimulation with synacthen. Clin Biochem. 2002;35(7):539–43.
5. Le Roux CW, Chapman GA, Kong WM, Dhillo WS, Jones J, AlaghbandZadeh J. Free cortisol index is better than serum total cortisol in determining hypothalamic-pituitary-adrenal status in patients undergoing surgery. J Clin Endocrinol Metab. 2003;88(5):2045–8.

Chapter 3
ACTH Stimulation Test for Late Onset (Nonclassic) 21-Hydroxylase Deficiency

Indication:	To evaluate for androgen excess in diagnosing non-classic CYP21A2 deficiency. If Basal 17-hydroxyprogesterone (17 OHP) <2 ng/ml, diagnosis is unlikely and ACTH stimulation may not be necessary [1, 2].
Preparation:	Women are best tested in the early follicular phase of the menstrual cycle. It is recommended to hold glucocorticoids for 24 h prior to testing to avoid any effect on 17 OH progesterone level.
Materials Needed:	Two (2) gold top tubes labeled as baseline and 60 minutes

---
Cortisol:
Gold top tube

17 OH Progesterone:
Gold top tube

Cortrosyn 250 mcg

Syringes/needles

Assay for 17 OHP:	Radioimmunoassay (RIA).
Interpretation:	With late onset 21-hydroxylase deficiency, the absolute value of 17-hydroxyprogesterone at 60 min sample is > 10 ng/dl [2, 3].

Caveats:

- Baseline androgen levels return to baseline after 8 weeks of discontinuation of oral contraceptive pills (OCP) [4].
- There is not enough data in regards to the effect of OCP on 17 OHP levels after ACTH stimulation.

© Springer International Publishing Switzerland 2015
A. B. Ergin et al., *The Cleveland Clinic Manual of Dynamic Endocrine Testing,*
DOI 10.1007/978-3-319-13048-4_3

Procedure: Completed as outpatient.

        1. Obtain baseline blood sample for (17 OHP) and cortisol.

        2. Give cortrosyn 250 mcg IM.

        3. At 60 min, obtain sample for (17 OHP) and cortisol.

Physician name and signature: _____

RN performing the procedure: _____

Additional orders by physician: _____

ACTH stimulation	Cortisol	17-OHP
Basal		
30 min		
60 min		

References

1. Azziz R, Zacur HA. 21-hydroxylase deficiency in female hyperandrogenism: screening and diagnosis. J Clin Endocrinol Metab. 1989;69(3):577–84.
2. Azziz R, Dewailly D, Owerbach D. Clinical review 56: nonclassic adrenal hyperplasia: current concepts. J Clin Endocrinol Metabo. 1994;78(4):810–5.
3. New MI, Lorenzen F, Lerner AJ, et al. Genotyping steroid 21-hydroxylase deficiency: hormonal reference data. J Clini Endocrinol Metabo. 1983;57(2):320–6.
4. Sanchez LA, Perez M, Centeno I, David M, Kahi D, Gutierrez E. Determining the time androgens and sex hormone-binding globulin take to return to baseline after discontinuation of oral contraceptives in women with polycystic ovary syndrome: a prospective study. Fertil Steril. 2007;87(3):712–4.

Chapter 4
Metyrapone Stimulation Test

Indication:	To evaluate HPA axis integrity. It is a sensitive alternative test to insulin tolerance test (ITT) in order to evaluate the adrenocorticotrophic hormone (ACTH) reserve.
Preparation:	The patient may eat and drink normally prior to the test.
Materials Needed:	

<table>
<tr><td>

ACTH:
Lavender top tube on ice

Transport Temperature:
Frozen;

Note: Separate plasma from cells ASAP

Cortisol and 11 deoxycortiol (DOC):
Gold top tube

</td><td>

Metyrapone po (30 mg/kg body weight, or 2 g for <70 kg, 2.5 g for 70 to 90 kg, and 3 g for >90 kg)

</td></tr>
</table>

Assay for Cortisol and ACTH:	Chemiluminescence Assay (CLIA).
Assay for 11 DOC:	LC-MS/MS.
Precautions:	Hypotension, nausea, vomiting, abdominal discomfort or cramping, and musculoskeletal pain in patients with adrenal insufficiency may happen. Metyrapone can also cause dizziness, sedation, and allergic rash.

© Springer International Publishing Switzerland 2015
A. B. Ergin et al., *The Cleveland Clinic Manual of Dynamic Endocrine Testing*,
DOI 10.1007/978-3-319-13048-4_4

Interpretation: Metyrapone blocks the conversion of 11-deoxy-cortisol to cortisol by CYP11B1 (11-beta-hydroxylase, P-450c11), the last step in the synthesis of cortisol, and induces a rapid fall of cortisol and stimulation of ACTH.

1. A normal response to the overnight single-dose test consists of [1–3]:
   - A serum cortisol concentration at 8 AM of less than 5 µg/dL (138 nmol/L) confirms adequate metyrapone blockade.
   - An 8 AM serum 11-DOC concentration >7 mcg/dL (>200 nmol/L).

2. A lack of achieving a serum 11-DOC concentration >7 mcg/dL in the presence of a serum cortisol >5 mcg/dL may be related to a lack of adequate 11 beta hydroxylase blockage. In such patients, the test needs to be repeated after taking higher dosage of metyrapone.

Caveats:

- The metyrapone test is the most sensitive method to detect partial defects in pituitary ACTH secretion [1, 3].
- Cortisol levels measured by conventional immunoassays can be falsely elevated by the interference of increased 11-deoxycortisol levels induced by metyrapone; Liquid chromatography tandem mass spectrometry steroid assays give the best results [4].
- Similar to ITT, the metyrapone test is not indicated for evaluation of patients suspected to have primary adrenal insufficiency. In such cases, measurement of morning serum cortisol, plasma ACTH level, or ACTH stimulation would be preferred.

Procedure: Completed as outpatient

1. Patient ingests metyrapone (30 mg/kg body weight, or 2 g for <70 kg, 2.5 g for 70–90 kg, and 3 g for >90 kg body weight at midnight/bedtime with a glass of milk or a small snack.
2. Serum 11-deoxycortisol, cortisol, and plasma ACTH are measured between 7:30 and 9:30 AM the next morning [1, 2].

References

1. Fiad TM, Kirby JM, Cunningham SK, McKenna TJ. The overnight single-dose metyrapone test is a simple and reliable index of the hypothalamic-pituitary-adrenal axis. Clin Endocrinol (Oxf). 1994;40(5):603–9.
2. Steiner H, Bähr V, Exner P, Oelkers P. Pituitary function tests: comparison of ACTH and 11-deoxy-cortisol responses in the metyrapone test and with the insulin hypoglycemia test. Exp Clinic Endocrinol Diabetes. 1994;102(01):33–8.
3. Gibney J, Healy M, Smith TP, McKenna TJ. A simple and cost-effective approach to assessment of pituitary adrenocorticotropin and growth hormone reserve: Combined use of the overnight metyrapone test and insulin-like growth factor-I standard deviation scores. J Clin Endocrinol Metab. 2008;93(10):3763–8.
4. Owen LJ, Halsall DJ, Keevil BG. Cortisol measurement in patients receiving metyrapone therapy. Ann Clin Biochem. 2010;47(6):573–5.

Chapter 5
Two Day Low Dose Dexamethasone Suppression Test

Indication:	To assess suppressibility of cortisol in patients with an equivocal screening test such as overnight 1 mg exametha-sone (dex) suppression test, 24 h urinary free cortisol, and/or late night salivary cortisol.
Preparation:	None.
Materials Needed:	Eight dexamethasone 0.5 mg tablets

<table>
<tr><td>Cortisol:
Gold top tube</td><td>One gold top tube for cortisol</td></tr>
</table>

Assay for Cortisol:	**Chemiluminescence Immunoassay (CLIA).**
Precautions:	None.
Interpretation:	Serum cortisol concentration > 1.4–1.8 µg/dl after 2 day low dose dex is strongly suggestive of Cushing's syndrome [1].

Caveats:

- Use of the 2 mg 2-day test has greater specificity at high sensitivity compared to the 1 mg overnight test. However, it requires more patience on the part of the patient [2, 3].
- We do not recommend 24 h urine cortisol measurement during 2 mg dexamethasone suppression test (DST) because measurement of serum cortisol concentration during the low dose dexamethasone test is simpler and more reliable than measurements of urinary steroids [3].
- Do not use this test if the patient is on estrogens which increase cortisol binding globulin (CBG) and falsely elevate cortisol levels [4].
- Drugs such as phenytoin, phenobarbital, phenobarbitone, carbamazepine, rifampicin, and alcohol induce hepatic enzymatic clearance of dexamethasone, mediated through CYP 3A4, thereby reducing the plasma dexamethasone concentrations and may be associated with a false positive result [5].

© Springer International Publishing Switzerland 2015
A. B. Ergin et al., *The Cleveland Clinic Manual of Dynamic Endocrine Testing*,
DOI 10.1007/978-3-319-13048-4_5

- To evaluate for false-positive and negative responses, some experts have advocated simultaneous measurement of both cortisol and dexamethasone during dexamethasone suppression tests to ensure adequate plasma dexamethasone concentrations.

Procedure: Completed as outpatient

1. Instruct patient to begin dexamethasone tablets. Patient takes one tablet every 6 h for a total of 8 doses (8 am, 2 pm, 8 pm, and 2 am). Some clinicians prefer a different schedule such as 6 am, 12 pm, 6 pm, and 12 am as a more convenient alternative. Studies were performed in the former schedule.
2. 6 h after the last dose, draw blood for cortisol (8 am).

   - Cortisol level at the end of the test: _____
   - Date and time of the cortisol:_____

Physician name and signature: _____

RN performing the procedure: _____

Additional orders by physician: _____

References

1. Isidori AM, Kaltsas GA, Mohammed S, et al. Discriminatory value of the low-dose dexamethasone suppression test in establishing the diagnosis and differential diagnosis of Cushing's syndrome. J Clin Endocrinol Metab. 2003;88(11):5299–306.
2. Kennedy L, Atkinson AB, Johnston H, Sheridan B, Hadden DR. Serum cortisol concentrations
   during low dose dexamethasone suppression test to screen for Cushing's syndrome. Br Med J
   Clin Res Ed. 1984;289(6453):1188–91.
3. Klose M, Lange M, Rasmussen AK, et al. Factors influencing the adrenocorticotropin test:
   role of contemporary cortisol assays, body composition, and oral contraceptive agents. J Clin
   Endocrinol Metab. 2007;92(4):1326–33.
4. Kyriazopoulou V, Vagenakis AG. Abnormal overnight dexamethasone suppression test in subjects receiving rifampicin therapy. J Clin Endocrinol Metab. 1992;75(1):315–7.
5. Meikle AW. Dexamethasone suppression tests: usefulness of simultaneous measurement of
   plasma cortisol and dexamethasone. Clin Endocrinol (Oxf). 1982;16(4):401–8.

Chapter 6
Combined CRH Dexamethasone Suppression Test

Indication:	To be able to distinguish Cushing's syndrome from pseudo-Cushing's states.
Preparation:	None.
Materials Needed:	Eight dexamethasone 0.5 mg tablets

Cortisol: Gold top tube	Two gold top tubes for cortisol, labeled baseline and post-dexamethasone

Assay for Cortisol:	Chemiluminescence Immunoassay (CLIA).
Precautions:	None.
Interpretation:	Serum cortisol concentration more than 1.4 mcg/dl at 15 min after Combined Dex-CRH test is suggestive of Cushing's syndrome [1].

Caveats:

- We do not recommend 24 h urine collection for cortisol because measurement of serum cortisol concentration during the low dose dexamethasone test is simpler than, and as accurate and reliable as, measurements of urinary steroids [2].
- The diagnostic accuracy of the dexamethasone-CRH test for Cushing's syndrome can be significantly greater than the accuracy of either the low-dose dexamethasone test or the CRH test alone [1].
- Do not use this test if the patient is on estrogens that increase cortisol-binding globulin (CBG) and falsely elevate cortisol levels [3].
- Drugs such as phenytoin, phenobarbitone, carbamazepine, rifampicin, and alcohol induce hepatic enzymatic clearance of dexamethasone, mediated through CYP 3A4, thereby reducing the plasma dexamethasone concentrations and may be associated with a false positive result [4].
- To evaluate for false-positive and negative responses, some experts have advocated simultaneous measurement of both cortisol and dexamethasone for these tests to ensure adequate plasma dexamethasone concentrations [5].

© Springer International Publishing Switzerland 2015
A. B. Ergin et al., *The Cleveland Clinic Manual of Dynamic Endocrine Testing*,
DOI 10.1007/978-3-319-13048-4_6

Procedure: Completed as outpatient.

1. Instruct patient to take one tablet every 6 h for a total of 8 doses (12 pm, 6 pm, 12 am, and 6 am).
2. Two hours after the last dose of dex (8 am), administer 100 mcg oCRH and draw blood for cortisol before and 15 min after oCRH administration.

- Cortisol level at the end of the test: _____
- Date and time of the cortisol: _____

Physician name and signature: _____

RN performing the procedure: _____

Additional orders by physician: _____

References

1. Yanovski JA, Cutler GBJ, Chrousos GP, Nieman LK. Corticotropin-releasing hormone stimulation following low-dose dexamethasone administration: a new test to distinguish cushing's syndrome from pseudo-Cushing's states. JAMA. 1993;269(17):2232–8.
2. Kennedy L, Atkinson AB, Johnston H, Sheridan B, Hadden DR. Serum cortisol concentrations during low dose dexamethasone suppression test to screen for Cushing's syndrome. Br Med J (Clin Res Ed). 1984;289(6453):1188–91.
3. Klose M, Lange M, Rasmussen AK, et al. Factors influencing the adrenocorticotropin test: role of contemporary cortisol assays, body composition, and oral contraceptive agents. J Clin Endocrinol Metab. 2007;92(4):1326–33.
4. Kyriazopoulou V, Vagenakis AG. Abnormal overnight dexamethasone suppression test in subjects receiving rifampicin therapy. J Clin Endocrinol Metab. 1992;75(1):315–7.
5. Meikle AW. Dexamethasone suppression tests: usefulness of simultaneous measurement of plasma cortisol and dexamethasone. Clin Endocrinol (Oxf). 1982;16(4):401–8.

Chapter 7
Overnight Low Dose Dexamethasone Suppression Test—1 mg

Indication:	To evaluate for Cushing's syndrome, to evaluate adrenal incidentaloma for subclinical Cushing's syndrome [1].
Preparation:	None.
Materials Needed:	Dexamethasone 1 mg po.
	One gold top tube for cortisol.
Precautions:	None.
Assay for Cortisol:	Chemiluminescence Immunoassay (CLIA).
Interpretation:	Normal response: Early morning cortisol < 1.8 µg/dL [2].
	Normal response in adrenal incidentaloma can be set at < 3–5 µg/dL if clinical significance and increased specificity are to be pursued.
	Serum dexamethasone level may be added to previously drawn cortisol sample if result is negative or equivocal.

Caveats:

- At the 1.8 µg/dL cutoff, the sensitivity is high (>95%) with specificity rates of 80%. Specificity increases to greater than 95% if the diagnostic threshold is raised to 5 µg/dL [3].
- Do not use this test if patient is on estrogens as they increase CBG resulting in falsely elevated cortisol levels [4].
- Drugs, such as phenytoin, phenobarbital, carbamazepine, rifampicin, and alcohol, induce hepatic enzymatic clearance of dexamethasone, mediated through CYP 3A4, thereby reducing the plasma dexamethasone concentrations and may be associated with a false positive result [5].

© Springer International Publishing Switzerland 2015
A. B. Ergin et al., *The Cleveland Clinic Manual of Dynamic Endocrine Testing*,
DOI 10.1007/978-3-319-13048-4_7

- To evaluate for false-positive and negative responses, some experts have advocated simultaneous measurement of both cortisol and dexamethasone during dexamethasone suppression tests to ensure adequate plasma dexamethasone concentrations [6].
- Patients with cyclic Cushing's syndrome may have a normal dexamethasone suppression test.

Procedure: Completed as outpatient.

1. Patient takes dexamethasone between 11 pm and midnight.
2. The next morning, the patient has serum cortisol drawn at laboratory at 8 am (fasting).

- Cortisol level at the end of the test: _____
- Date and time of the cortisol: _____

Physician name and signature: _____

RN performing the procedure: _____

Additional orders by physician: _____

References

1. Kannan S, Remer EM, Hamrahian AH. Evaluation of patients with adrenal incidentalomas. Curr Opin Endocrinol Diabetes Obes. 2013;20(3):161–9.
2. Wood PJ, Barth JH, Freedman DB, Perry L, Sheridan B. Evidence for the low dose dexamethasone suppression test to screen for Cushing's syndrome—recommendations for a protocol for biochemistry laboratories. Ann Clin Biochem. 1997;34(Pt 3):222–9.
3. Martin NM, Dhillo WS, Meeran K. The dexamethasone-suppressed corticotropin-releasing hormone stimulation test and the desmopressin test to distinguish Cushing's syndrome from pseudo-Cushing's states. Clin Endocrinol (Oxf). 2007;67(3):476.
4. Klose M, Lange M, Rasmussen AK, Skakkebaek NE, Hilsted L, Haug E, et al. Factors influencing the adrenocorticotropin test: role of contemporary cortisol assays, body composition, and oral contraceptive agents. J Clin Endocrinol Metab. 2007;92(4):1326–33.
5. Kyriazopoulou V, Vagenakis AG. Abnormal overnight dexamethasone suppression test in subjects receiving rifampicin therapy. J Clin Endocrinol Metab. 1992;75(1):315–7.
6. Meikle AW. Dexamethasone suppression tests: usefulness of simultaneous measurement of plasma cortisol and dexamethasone. Clin Endocrinol (Oxf). 1982;16(4):401–8.

Chapter 8
Overnight High Dose Dexamethasone Suppression Test—8 mg

Indication:	1. To help differentiate Cushing's disease from ectopic ACTH syndrome (EAS) in patients with ACTH-dependent Cushing's syndrome.
	2. To help differentiate Cushing's disease from adrenal Cushing's in patients with low normal plasma ACTH levels.
Preparation:	Overnight fast is recommended.
Materials Needed:	Dexamethasone 8 mg.
Precautions:	None.
Assay for Cortisol:	Chemiluminescence Immunoassay (CLIA).
Interpretation:	The basis for the high-dose suppression tests is the fact that ACTH secretion in Cushing's disease is only relatively resistant to glucocorticoid negative feedback inhibition. Cortisol levels will not suppress normally with overnight 1 mg but will suppress with 8 mg high dose dexamethasone suppression test [1].

- Serum cortisol concentration at 8 am is <5 mcg/dL (140 nmol/L) in most patients with Cushing's disease, and is usually undetectable in normal individuals.
- A more than 50% decrease in cortisol on the day after taking 8-mg dexamethasone supports a diagnosis of Cushing's disease. A 77–92% sensitivity and 57–100% specificity is reported in different studies [2–4]. More stringent criteria >68% and >80% suppression of cortisol have been suggested by some groups to improve its diagnostic specificity [2].

© Springer International Publishing Switzerland 2015
A. B. Ergin et al., *The Cleveland Clinic Manual of Dynamic Endocrine Testing*,
DOI 10.1007/978-3-319-13048-4_8

- A lack of suppression of cortisol by more than 50% during the high-dose dexamethasone suppression test (DST) in patients with low normal ACTH levels (5–20 pg/ml) suggests an adrenal etiology because adrenal tumors do not depend on ACTH for cortisol secretion.

Caveats:

- Dexamethasone levels can be measured to assure compliance and a lack of increased metabolism.
- Drugs, such as phenytoin, phenobarbitone, carbamazepine, rifampicin, and alcohol, induce hepatic enzymatic clearance of dexamethasone, mediated through CYP 3A4, thereby reducing the plasma dexamethasone concentrations and may be associated with a false positive result [5].
- To evaluate for false-positive and negative responses, some experts have advocated simultaneous measurement of both cortisol and dexamethasone for these tests to ensure adequate plasma dexamethasone concentrations [6].
- A more than 50% decrease in cortisol during the high-dose dexamethasone suppression test, and a more than 50% increase in ACTH after CRH stimulation has a 98% positive predictive value for Cushing's disease. *However, 18–65% of patients with Cushing's disease lacked a response to one or both tests* [7, 8].

Procedure: Completed as outpatient.

1. Patient has serum cortisol drawn between 8–9 am, then takes dexamethasone that evening at 11 pm.
2. The next morning, the cortisol is drawn again between 8–9 am while fasting [1].

   • Cortisol level at baseline before dexamathasone: _____

   • Cortisol level at the end of the test: _____

   • Date and time of the cortisol: _____

Physician name and signature: _____

References

1. Liddle GW. Tests of pituitary-adrenal suppressibility in the diagnosis of Cushing's syndrome. Endocrinologist. 1960;20:1539.
2. Bruno OD, Rossi MA, Contreras LN, et al. Nocturnal high-dose dexamethasone suppression test in the aetiological diagnosis of Cushing's syndrome. Acta Endocrinol (Copenh). 1985;109(2):158–62.
3. Dichek HL, Nieman LK, Oldfield EH, Pass HI, Malley JD, Cutler GB Jr. A comparison of the standard high dose dexamethasone suppression test and the overnight 8-mg dexamethasone suppression test for the differential diagnosis of adrenocorticotropin-dependent Cushing's syndrome. J Clin Endocrinol Metab. 1994;78(2):418–22.
4. Tyrrell JB, Findling JW, Aron DC, Fitzgerald PA, Forsham PH. An overnight high-dose dexamethasone suppression test for rapid differential diagnosis of Cushing's syndrome. Ann Intern Med. 1986;104(2):180–6.
5. Kyriazopoulou V, Vagenakis AG. Abnormal overnight dexamethasone suppression test in subjects receiving rifampicin therapy. J Clin Endocrinol Metab. 1992;75(1):315–7.
6. Meikle AW. Dexamethasone suppression tests: usefulness of simultaneous measurement of plasma cortisol and dexamethasone. Clin Endocrinol (Oxf). 1982;16(4):401–8.
7. Nieman LK, Chrousos GP, Oldfield EH, Avgerinos PC, Cutler GB Jr, Loriaux DL. The ovine corticotropin-releasing hormone stimulation test and the dexamethasone suppression test in the differential diagnosis of Cushing's syndrome. Ann Intern Med. 1986;105(6):862–7.
8. Nieman, et al. Evaluation and treatment of Cushing's syndrome. Am J Med. 2005;118:1340–6.

Chapter 9
Ovine Corticotropin-Releasing Hormone (oCRH) Stimulation Test

Indication:	To differentiate Cushing's disease from ectopic and adrenal Cushing's syndrome.
Patient Preparation:	Patient to fast or abstain from eating for at least 4 h before the test since there may be a physiologic increase in cortisol levels after a meal [1].
Pregnancy Category C:	There is positive evidence of human fetal risk based on adverse reaction data from investigational or marketing experience or studies in humans, but potential benefits may warrant use of the drug in pregnant women despite potential risks.
Materials Needed:	1. Six lavender-top (EDTA) tubes on ice for ACTH (adrenocorticotrophic hormone) labeled − 15, 0, 15, 30, 45, and 60 min.
	2. Six gold top tubes for cortisol labeled − 15, 0, 15, 30, 45, and 60 min.
	3. ACTHREL (ovine CRH) 1 mcg/kg to be administered over 30 s (maximum dose of 100 mcg).
	4. IV line catheter/syringes/needles.

ACTH Lavender-top tube (**on ice**), 1 ml Method: Electrochemiluminescence immunoassay (ECLIA)

Cortisol:
Gold top tube, 1 ml, Chemiluminescence Immunoassay (CLIA)

© Springer International Publishing Switzerland 2015
A. B. Ergin et al., *The Cleveland Clinic Manual of Dynamic Endocrine Testing*,
DOI 10.1007/978-3-319-13048-4_9

Precautions: Monitor blood pressure and pulse rate if the patient is
                                     symptomatic, since episodes of hypotension and tachy-
                                     cardia have rarely been reported. Flushing of face,
                                     neck, and upper chest and the urge to take a deep breath
                                     have also been noted. All signs and symptoms could
                                     be reduced by administering the drug over 30 s instead
                                     of bolus injection. The use of a heparin solution to
                                     maintain IV cannula patency during the corticotrophin-
                                     releasing hormone (CRH test) is not recommended.
                                     An interaction between CRH and heparin may cause a
                                     hypotensive reaction (see drug label).

Interpretation:

- Cushing's syndrome due to pituitary tumors causing Cushing's disease usually responds to CRH with increased ACTH
  and/or cortisol; whereas ectopic ACTH-secreting tumors
  and adrenal tumors usually do not.
- More than 35–50 % increase in the basal plasma ACTH concentration or a more than 20 % increase in the basal serum
  cortisol concentration suggests Cushing's disease [2, 3].

Caveats:

1. Approximately 8 % of patients with Cushing's disease do not respond to CRH
   with no appreciable increase in peripheral plasma ACTH or serum cortisol concentrations [4].
2. CRH test is used to differentiate Cushing's disease from Adrenal Cushing's when
   the ACTH level is in the indeterminate range (for most assays, 5–20 pg/mL).
3. Occasional patients with ectopic ACTH syndrome or primary adrenal disease
   may respond to CRH. In such patients, a lack of completely suppressed hypothalamic–pituitary axis has been suggested as the underlying etiology. A more than
   50 % decrease in cortisol during the overnight high-dose dexamethasone suppression test, and a more than 50 % increase in ACTH after the CRH stimulation
   has 98 % positive predictive value for Cushing's disease. However, up to 30 % of
   patients with Cushing's disease fail one of the two tests [5].

CRH Stimulation Test Procedure: Completed as outpatient.

1. Patient to fast after midnight or abstain from eating for at least 4 h.
2. Check the materials needed in the first page.
3. Establish IV line. Flush with saline only. Do not use heparin.
4. Allow patient to rest for 30 min.
5. Draw baseline samples for ACTH and cortisol at -15 and 0 min.
6. Give CRH slowly IV over 30–60 s.
7. Draw blood samples at 15, 30, 45, and 60 min for cortisol and ACTH.

Patient name: _____

Physician name and signature: _____

RN performing the procedure: _____

Additional orders by physician: _____

CRH test	-15 min	0 min (baseline)	15 min	30 min	45 min	60 min
Cortisol						
ACTH						

References

1. Ishizuka B, Quigley ME, Yen SS. Pituitary hormone release in response to food ingestion: evidence for neuroendocrine signals from gut to brain. J Clin Endocrinol Metab. 1983;57(6):1111–6.
2. Nieman LK, Oldfield EH, Wesley R, Chrousos GP, Loriaux DL, Cutler GB Jr. A simplified morning ovine corticotropin-releasing hormone stimulation test for the differential diagnosis of adrenocorticotropin-dependent Cushing's syndrome. J Clin Endocrinol Metab. 1993;77(5):1308–12.
3. Reimondo G, Paccotti P, Minetto M, et al. The corticotrophin-releasing hormone test is the most reliable noninvasive method to differentiate pituitary from ectopic ACTH secretion in Cushing's syndrome. Clin Endocrinol (Oxf). 2003;58(6):718–24.
4. Dickstein G, DeBold CR, Gaitan D, et al. Plasma corticotropin and cortisol responses to ovine corticotropin-releasing hormone (CRH), arginine vasopressin (AVP), CRH plus AVP, and CRH plus metyrapone in patients with Cushing's disease. J Clin Endocrinol Metab. 1996;81(8):2934–41.
5. Nieman LK, Chrousos GP, Oldfield EH, Avgerinos PC, Cutler GB, Jr, Loriaux DL. The ovine corticotropin-releasing hormone stimulation test and the dexamethasone suppression test in the differential diagnosis of Cushing's syndrome. Ann Intern Med. 1986;105(6):862–7.

Chapter 10
Insulin Tolerance Test (ITT)

Indication:	This test is performed to evaluate patients with suspected hypothalamic-pituitary-adrenal (HPA) axis or growth hormone (GH) axis deficiency. Hypoglycemia causes a major stress response, with an increase in plasma ACTH, serum cortisol, and growth hormone. Insulin Tolerance Test (ITT) is considered the gold standard test to evaluate the integrity of HPA.
Contraindication:	History of coronary artery disease, seizure disorder, or stroke. Age more than 65 is a relative contraindication.
Preparation:	NPO except water after midnight and during test
	Confirm patient medications and NPO status with a physician prior to proceeding.
Materials Needed:	A syringe containing 50% glucose solution should be at the bedside.

Cortisol:
Gold top tube
GH: Gold top
tube
Glucose:
Gray top tube
Assays: Cortisol: CLIA GH:
Immunoenzymatic

Insulin—confirm dose with a physician
Crackers/juice/soda
Glucose monitor
Twenty-one (21) gold top tubes

Precautions:	Do not leave the patient unattended since hypoglycemia is expected.
	A physician must be available in the walking distance from the room where the ITT is performed.

© Springer International Publishing Switzerland 2015
A. B. Ergin et al., *The Cleveland Clinic Manual of Dynamic Endocrine Testing*,
DOI 10.1007/978-3-319-13048-4_10

Interpretation:

- A cortisol level <500 nmol/L (18 μg/dL) is consistent with an abnormal HPA axis [1].
- A serum growth hormone <5 ng/ml (5 mcg/L) is consistent with severe growth hormone deficiency (96% sensitivity and 92% specificity) [2]. To obtain 95% specificity, a lower peak serum GH cut point at 3 μg/ml (3 ng/ml) may be used [2].

Caveats:

- The test should be performed by an experienced clinician
- To be able to interpret test results, patients should achieve a glucose level <2.2 nmol/L (40 mg/dL) associated with symptoms of hypoglycemia including headache, palpitation, diaphoresis and mental fogginess.
- The test is not indicated for evaluation of patients suspected to have primary adrenal insufficiency.
- Once hypoglycemia is developed, providing intravenous 50% glucose solution or juice does not alter the result of the test.

Insulin Tolerance Test Procedure:

1. Establish hep-lock.
2. Draw baseline, timed samples after 30 min of patient rest for GH, cortisol, and glucose
3. Inject regular insulin IV in a single push as ordered by a physician and 10 cc saline flush following insulin.
4. Note the time of insulin injection.
5. Obtain samples for GH, cortisol, and glucose at 15, 30, 45, 60, 90, and 120 min after insulin injection.
6. The symptoms of hypoglycemia may be mild in patients with long standing secondary adrenal insufficiency or panhypopituitarism. In such patients close monitoring of the patient is required for subtle changes in mental status.
7. Provide the patient with juice and cracker at the end of the test. Patients should have two consecutive blood glucose levels >4 mmol/L (70 mg/dl), 15 min apart before leaving the testing area. Advise the patient to eat a meal containing protein before leaving the hospital.

Guidelines for Initial and Repeat Insulin Orders: The standard dose is generally 0.15 unit/kg (0.1 unit/kg for a patient with known secondary adrenal insufficiency when he/she is being evaluated for GH deficiency). In patients with obesity or suspected insulin resistance, the dose may be increased up to 0.25 unit/kg.

*Redosing may be necessary if BG does not decrease by 30 min. If BG is not less than 45 mg/dl at 30 min, administer another dose of 50–100% of the initial dose based on the BG and the decline from baseline value.

Patient label: _____

Insulin dose initial:_____

RN performing the procedure:_____

Ordering provider's signature:_____ Date:_____

ITT	Baseline	15 min	30 min	45 min	60 min	90 min	120 min
BG							
Cortisol							
GH							

References

1. Dorin RI, Qualls CR, Crapo LM. Diagnosis of adrenal insufficiency. Ann Intern Med. 2003;139(3):194–204.
2. Biller BMK, Samuels MH, Zagar A, et al. Sensitivity and specificity of six tests for the diagnosis of adult GH deficiency. J Clin Endocrinol Metab. 2002;87(5):2067–9.

Chapter 11
Glucagon Stimulation Test for GHD (GST)

Indication:	1. In order to evaluate patients with suspected growth hormone (GH) deficiency.
	2. In order to assess growth hormone reserve when insulin tolerance test or growth hormone-releasing hormone (GHRH)–arginine tests are contraindicated, not preferred, or not available.
Contraindication:	Malnourishment, pheochromocytoma, or insulinoma [5].
Preparation:	Nil per os (NPO) except water after midnight and during test
Materials needed:	Nine gold top tubes, glucagon

> **GH:**
> 2 ml Gold top tube

Assay for GH:	Immunoenzymatic
Precautions:	Nausea (30%), vomiting/retching (10%), and headaches (10%) may occur during and after the test. (Administration of intravenous antiemetics can be considered.) Late hypoglycemia may rarely occur (patients should be advised to eat small and frequent meals after the completion of the test) [5].
Interpretation:	In adults with growth hormone deficiency (GHD), peak GH levels fail to rise above 3 ng/mL (sensitivity 97–100% and specificity 88–100%) [1, 2]. Preliminary results of ongoing studies suggest lower cutoff values for diagnosis of severe GH deficiency.

© Springer International Publishing Switzerland 2015
A. B. Ergin et al., *The Cleveland Clinic Manual of Dynamic Endocrine Testing,*
DOI 10.1007/978-3-319-13048-4_11

Caveats:

- It is not known whether testing using the GST in subjects with diabetes is valid, since only a small number of patients with diabetes have been included in clinical studies [3, 5].
- Unlike the GHRH–arginine test, significant correlation between body mass index (BMI) and peak GH response to the GST was observed in some but not all the studies [2].
- It is still not clear whether the ideal timing of the GST is 3 versus 4 hour, and continuing the test for 4 hour may be advisable, at least until there are more definitive data available [4].

Procedure [5]:

1. Ensure patient fasts from midnight.

2. Weigh patient and document the weight.

3. Insert intravenous cannula (hep-lock) for intravenous access between 8 and 9 a.m.

4. Administer glucagon intramuscularly 1 mg (1.5 mg if patient weighs more than 90 kg) [1]. Confirm the medication doses with physician.

5. Monitor blood pressure (BP) and point-of-care (POC) blood sugar every 30 min during test if patient is symptomatic.

6. Discontinue hep-lock.

7. Collect serum GH and capillary blood glucose levels at 0, 30, 60, 90,120, 150, 180, 210, and 240 min [5].

Patient label: _____

Documentation for medication orders: _____

Ordering provider's signature: _____ Date: _____

Glucagon stim test (min)	Time	Growth hormone	BG POC
Basal (0)			
30			
60			
90			
120			
150			
180			
210			
240			

BG POC blood glucose point of care

References

1. Conceicao FL, da Costa e Silva A, Leal Costa AJ, Vaisman M. Glucagon stimulation test for the diagnosis of GH deficiency in adults. J Endocrinol Invest. 2003;26(11):1065–70.
2. Gomez JM, Espadero RM, EscobarJimenez F, et al. Growth hormone release after glucagon as a reliable test of growth hormone assessment in adults. Clin Endocrinol (Oxf). 2002;56(3): 329–34.
3. Ogawa N. Stimulation tests of human growth hormone secretion by insulin, lysine vasopressin, pyrogen, and glucagon. Acta Med Okayama. 1974;28(3):181–97.
4. Orme SM, Price A, et al. Comparison of the diagnostic utility of the simplified and standard i.m. glucagon stimulation test (IMGST). Clin Endocrinol (Oxf) 1998;49(6):773–8.
5. Yuen KC. Glucagon stimulation testing in assessing for adult growth hormone deficiency: Current status and future perspectives. ISRN Endocrinol. 2011;2011:608056.

Chapter 12
GHRH–Arginine GH Stimulation Test

Indication:	1. In order to evaluate patients with suspected GH deficiency
	2. In order to assess growth hormone reserve when insulin tolerance test is contraindicated/not preferred
Preparation:	NPO except water after midnight and during test
	Confirm testing with physician prior to proceeding.
Materials needed:	Five gold top tubes

GH:
Gold top tube

GHRH

Arginine

Confirm the medication doses with physician.

Assay for GH:	GH:Immunoenzymatic Assay
Precautions:	Facial flushing occurs immediately after administration of GHRH in about half of the patients. Paresthesias, nausea, and abnormal taste sensation occur in 5–10% patients [1].
Interpretation:	Serum growth hormone (<4.1 ng/mL) confirms the diagnosis of growth hormone deficiency with 95% sensitivity and 91% specificity compared to 96% sensitivity and 92% specificity of ITT (GH <5.1 ng/mL) in patients with BMI >30 [1].

© Springer International Publishing Switzerland 2015
A. B. Ergin et al., *The Cleveland Clinic Manual of Dynamic Endocrine Testing,*
DOI 10.1007/978-3-319-13048-4_12

Suggested GH cut-offs based on BMI [2]

BMI <25 kg/m^2	Peak GH <11.5 mcg/L
BMI 25–30 kg/m^2	Peak GH <8 mcg/L
BMI >30 kg/m^2	Peak GH <4.1 mcg/L

Caveats:

- The ARG–GHRH test performs equally well in diagnosing GHD, indicating that it provides an ideal alternative to the ITT [1].
- This test can give a falsely normal GH response in patients with GHD of hypothalamic origin, e.g., those having received irradiation of the hypothalamic-pituitary region because GHRH directly stimulates the pituitary [3].
- Decreased responsiveness to stimulation tests such as GHRH, ITT, and ARG–GHRH has been demonstrated in subjects with obesity and/or abdominal adiposity [4].

Procedure: Completed as outpatient.

1. Check the *Dynamic Testing Order Sheet.*
2. Establish hep-lock.
3. Draw baseline, timed samples after 30 min of patient rest for GH
4. Inject 1 mcg/kg of GHRH IV in a single push followed immediately by 0.5 g/kg (to a maximum of 30 g) of arginine HCl IV infusion over 30 min as ordered by physician and followed by 10 cc saline flush.
5. Note the time of GHRH and arginine injection.
6. Obtain samples for GH at: 30, 60, 90, and 120 min.

Patient label:_____

Documentation for medication orders:_____

Ordering provider's signature: _____Date:_____

GHRH–arginine test	Time	Growth hormone
Basal (after 30 min of rest)		
Post-30 min		
Post-60 min		
Post-90 min		
Post-120 min		

References

1. Biller BMK, Samuels MH, Zagar A, et al. Sensitivity and specificity of six tests for the diagnosis of adult GH deficiency. J Clin Endocrinol Metab. 2002;87(5):2067–9.
2. Corneli G, Di Somma C, Baldelli R, et al. The cut-off limits of the GH response to GH-releasing hormone-arginine test related to body mass index. Eur J Endocrinol. 2005;153(2):257–64.
3. Darzy KH, Aimaretti G, Wieringa G, Gattamaneni HR, Ghigo E, Shalet SM. The usefulness of the combined growth hormone (GH)-releasing hormone and arginine stimulation test in the diagnosis of radiation-induced GH deficiency is dependent on the post-irradiation time interval. J Clin Endocrinol Metab. 2003;88(1):95–102.
4. Vizner B, Reiner Z, Sekso M. Effect of l-dopa on growth hormone, glucose, insulin, and cortisol response in obese subjects. Exp Clin Endocrinol. 1983;81(1):41–8.

Chapter 13
Growth Hormone Suppression Test (Post-Glucose Administration)

Indication:	To establish the diagnosis of acromegaly when there is modest elevation of IGF-1 (<2-fold upper limit of normal) with absent or equivocal clinical features [1]
Preparation:	10 h fasting
Materials Needed:	Glucose drink 75 g

Glucose:
Grey top tube

Growth hormone:
Gold top tube

Five (5) Gold top tubes labeled baseline, 30, 60, 90 and 120 minutes

Four (4) grey top tubes labeled 30, 60, 90 and 120 minutes

Saline lock/ 22 G angiocath

Assay for GH:	Immunoenzymatic assay
Precautions:	Patients may complain of nausea.
Interpretation:	Diagnosis of acromegaly: Using ultrasensitive assays, a GH suppression to <0.4 ng/ml is considered the gold standard test to rule out acromegaly [2]. The GH cutoff value may vary based on the assay used. The authors use a GH cutoff value <0.2 ng/mL as a normal response, using a immunoenzymatic assay at Cleveland Clinic [1].

A GH level <1 ng/mL early after surgery, in the absence of presurgical usage of somatostatin analogs, predict long-term remission [3].

© Springer International Publishing Switzerland 2015
A. B. Ergin et al., *The Cleveland Clinic Manual of Dynamic Endocrine Testing,*
DOI 10.1007/978-3-319-13048-4_13

Caveats:

- Endocrinologists should be familiar with the assays used in their laboratories, including the expected normal nadir GH level after oral glucose e [4].
- Elevated IGF-1 levels more than twice the upper limit of normal in patients with clinical features suggestive of an underlying acromegaly, are usually sufficient to establish the diagnosis [1].
- Failure of adequate suppression or a paradoxical rise in GH level can be seen in starvation, anorexia nervosa, and chronic renal failure, but these conditions are typically associated with low IGF-1 levels.
- GH levels during OGTT have not been well studied in patients with diabetes mellitus, and in those on estrogen . In the authors' experience, patients with diabetes who are not poorly controlled achieve GH levels during OGTT similar to those without DM [5].
- A paradoxical GH secretary response to glucose may be seen in premature infants, children of tall stature, and adolescents [6].

Procedure: Completed as outpatient.

1. Establish saline lock.
2. Check POC BG.
3. Draw baseline growth hormone.
4. Give glucose 75 g orally (glucose drink).
5. Draw glucose and growth hormone levels at 30, 60, 90, and 120 min [7].
6. (Include insulin levels at baseline, 30, 60, 90, and 120 min only if requested).

Patient label: _____

Physician name and signature: _____

RN performing the procedure: _____

Additional orders by physician: _____

GH suppression test	Baseline	30 min	60 min	90 min	120 min
Glucose					
GH					

References

1. Subbarayan SK, Fleseriu M, Gordon MB, et al. Serum IGF-1 in the diagnosis of acromegaly and the profile of patients with elevated IGF-1 but normal glucose-suppressed growth hormone. Endocr Pract. 2012;18(6):817–25.
2. Katznelson L, Atkinson JL, Cook DM, Ezzat SZ, Hamrahian AH, Miller KK. American association of clinical endocrinologists medical guidelines for clinical practice for the diagnosis and treatment of acromegaly-2011 update. Endocr Pract. 2011;17:1–44.
3. Minuto F, Resmini E, Boschetti M, et al. Assessment of disease activity in acromegaly by means of a single blood sample: Comparison of the 120th minute postglucose value with spontaneous GH secretion and with the IGF system. Clin Endocrinol (Oxf). 2004;61(1):138–44.
4. Melmed S, Casanueva F, Cavagnini F, et al. Consensus statement: Medical management of acromegaly. Eur J Endocrinol . 2005;153(6):737–40.
5. Dobri GA, Faiman C, Kennedy L, et al. Is the GH Nadir value during OGTT reliable in diagnosing acromegaly in patients with altered glucose metabolism? Poster Board SAT-128, Endo 2013. https://Endo.confex.com/endo/2013endo/webprogram/Paper7607.html.
6. Hattori N, Shimatsu A, Kato Y, et al. Growth hormone responses to oral glucose loading measured by highly sensitive enzyme immunoassay in normal subjects and patients with glucose intolerance and acromegaly. J Clin Endocrinol Metab. 1990;70(3):771–6.
7. Earll JM, Sparks LL, Forsham PH. Glucose suppression of serum growth hormone in the diagnosis of acromegaly. JAMA. 1967;201(8):628–30.

Chapter 14
Clonidine Suppression Test

Indication:	To evaluate for pheochromocytoma when plasma norepinephrine (NE) is 1000–2000 pg/ml and/or plasma normetanephrine (NM) elevation that is less than four times the upper limit of normal reference range. The test is performed to distinguish patients with pheochromocytoma from those with elevated plasma norepinephrine and normetanephrine levels from other etiologies.
Patient Preparation:	Fasting for 10 h [1].
Materials Needed:	Clonidine 0.3 mg (0.3 mg dose is recommended for patients with 60–80 kg body weight, adjusted dose 4.3 µg/kg, maximum 0.5 mg) [1–2]
	4 Lavender-top (EDTA) tube for baseline and 3 h time points.

Plasma metanephrines
Lavender-top
(EDTA) tube,
1 ml
Method: liquid
chromatography/
tandem mass
spectrometry
(LC/MS-MS)

Plasma Catecholamines:
Lavender-top
(EDTA) tube or
Green-top (heparin) tube, 3 ml
Method: High-pressure liquid
chromatography
(HPLC)
Keep samples
ON ICE

Precautions: Sustained hypotension may occur. Keep patient supine
                          throughout testing.

                          Patients may experience dry mouth or drowsiness [1]

Interpretation: Criteria for diagnosis of pheochromocytoma: 3 h after cloni-
                          dine; one of the criteria below confirms the diagnosis [3]:

                          1. Lack of suppression of NM more than 40% and NM
                             above upper limit of normal (Sensitivity (sn): 96%,
                             specificity (sp):100%)
                          2. Elevated plasma concentration of NM above upper nor-
                             mal reference range (sn: 96%, sp: 96%)
                          3. Elevated plasma concentration of NE above upper nor-
                             mal reference range (Sn: 71% and sp: 94%)
                          4. Less than 50% NE suppression (sn 81%, sp: 82%)

Caveats:

1. The test may be associated with hypotension in patients with normal blood
   pressure.
2. In most patients careful evaluation of plasma and urinary metanephrines and
   catecholamines of interfering drugs, and their correlation with imaging studies
   (if available) may obviate the need for a clonidine suppression test.
3. Medications to avoid prior to clonidine suppression test: phenoxybenzamine and
   tricyclic antidepressants. Selective Alpha 1 -adrenergic blockers do not interfere with the test and can be used to control hypertension [3–4]. Beta blockers,
   calcium channel blockers, and diuretics may affect plasma norepinephrine levels,
   but do not have any significant effect on normetanephrine levels [3–4].
4. Patients who have relatively low baseline catecholamines levels (<1000 pg/ml)
   may have high false positive test results if criteria less than 50% reduction on
   norepinephrine levels is used [3, 5].
5. Measurement of plasma normetanephrine levels during clonidine suppression
   test provide better diagnostic sensitivity and specificity compared to plasma norepinephrine levels [3].
6. The clonidine suppression test cannot be used to evaluate patients with an
   elevated plasma metanephrine fraction since clonidine has a minimal effect on
   metanephrine levels. Similarly, the clonidine suppression test cannot be used
   in patients with rare dopamine secreting pheochromocytomas or measurement
   of plasma methoxytyramine (when commercially available); plasma or urinary
   dopamine may be used in such patients.

Procedure:

1. Patient to fast for 10 h prior to the test
2. Establish a heplock.
3. The patient should be relaxed and comfortable in the bed.
4. Allow patient to rest undisturbed 20 to 30 min.
5. Check blood pressure. If blood pressure is <120/80 mmHg, need to use caution and may consider postponing the test.
6. Draw baseline plasma norepinephrine and plasma normetanephrine. For plasma metanephrines, draw blood in chilled lavender-top (EDTA) tube. Invert to mix with preservatives (the whole blood sample may be kept refrigerated at 4 °C for as long as 2 h before centrifugation, if necessary). For plasma catecholamines, draw blood in lavender-top (EDTA) tube or green-top (heparin) tube. Invert to mix with preservatives. Place the blood sample on ice but do not freeze it. The time between blood collection and the preparation of plasma should be less than 1 h. If the time exceeds 1 h, catecholamine values increase (when blood is kept at 4 °C) or decrease (when left at 20 °C). **Submit separate specimens for baseline and 3 h time point**.
7. Give Clonidine 0.3 mg orally with 250 ml of water (0.3 mg dose is recommended for patients 60–80 kg body weight, adjusted dose 4.3 µg/kg, maximum 0.5 mg).
8. Three hours after ingestion of clonidine, record blood pressure and draw blood samples for plasma norepinephrine and plasma normetanephrine (**keep on ice, but do not freeze it**).

Patient label _____

Clonidine dose: _____

Ordering Provider's Signature: _____ Date_____

	Norepinephrine	Normetanephrine	Blood pressure/Heart rate
Baseline			
3 h			

References

1. Bravo EL, Tarazi RC, Fouad FM, Vidt DG, Gifford RW,Jr. Clonidine-suppression test: a useful aid in the diagnosis of pheochromocytoma. N Engl J Med. 1981;305(11):623–6. (NIH Clonidine suppression test protocol at https://science.nichd.nih.gov/confluence/download/attachments/23920688/Clonidine+suppression+test+v2.doc).
2. Eisenhofer G, Goldstein DS, Walther MM, et al. Biochemical diagnosis of pheochromocytoma: how to distinguish true- from false-positive test results. J Clin Endocrinol Metab. 2003;88(6):2656–66.
3. Sjoberg RJ, Simcic KJ, Kidd GS. The clonidine suppression test for pheochromocytoma. A review of its utility and pitfalls. Arch Intern Med. 1992;152(6):1193–7.
4. Bravo EL, Gifford RW,Jr. Current concepts. pheochromocytoma: diagnosis, localization and management. N Engl J Med. 1984;311(20):1298–1303.
5. Proye C, Fossati P, Fontaine P, et al. Dopamine-secreting pheochromocytoma: an unrecognized entity? classification of pheochromocytomas according to their type of secretion. Surgery. 1986;100(6):1154–62.

Chapter 15
Intravenous Saline Suppression Test

Indication:	Confirmatory test for suspected primary aldosteronism.
Preparation:	Keep patient supine x 30 min prior to the test start.
Materials needed:	Two lavender-top and 2 light green-top tubes, labeled baseline and at 4 h.

> **Aldosterone:**
> Lavender top

Normal saline: 2 L.

IV infusion set.

Heplock/syringes/needle.

Assay for Aldosterone:	Enzymatic radioimmunoassay (RIA).
Precautions:	Do not perform this test in patients with severe uncontrolled hypertension, renal insufficiency, cardiac insufficiency, cardiac arrhythmia, or severe hypokalemia.
Interpretation:	Postinfusion plasma aldosterone levels <5 ng/dL make the diagnosis of primary aldosteronism (PA) unlikely, and levels >10 ng/dL are a very probable sign of PA. Values between 5 and 10 ng/dL are indeterminate [1–3].

Caveats:

- Stop all potassium sparing and potassium wasting diuretics for 4 weeks. Stop beta-adrenergic blockers, central alpha-2 agonists (e.g., clonidine, alpha-methyl-dopa), non-steroidal anti-inflammatory drugs, angiotensin-converting enzyme inhibitors, angiotensin receptor blockers, renin inhibitors, dihydropyridine calcium channel antagonists for 2 weeks [1]. Blood pressure can be controlled with verapamil, prazosin, doxazosin, terazosin, or hydralazine in the meantime [1].
- Potassium levels should be corrected prior to the test [1].

© Springer International Publishing Switzerland 2015
A. B. Ergin et al., *The Cleveland Clinic Manual of Dynamic Endocrine Testing*,
DOI 10.1007/978-3-319-13048-4_15

- When aldosterone levels are in the indeterminate category, other confirmatory tests should be performed, such as oral salt loading test or captopril challenge test [3]. Although Fludrocortisone suppression test has more diagnostic accuracy, it requires hospitalization.
- Measuring plasma renin activity (PRA) and/or cortisol does not improve the diagnostic accuracy performance of the test [4].
- In patients with severe uncontrolled hypertension (BP > 180/100 mmHg), delaying the test till better BP control is achieved, or proceeding with the Captopril challenge test may be considered.

Procedure:

1. Patient must remain supine throughout test and 30 min prior to start of the test.
2. Establish Heplock.
3. Obtain baseline blood sample for aldosterone and Basic metabolic panel (BMP).
4. Infuse 2 L NS over 4 h.
5. Monitor patient for congestive heart failure (CHF) (tachycardia, dyspnea, leg edema) and blood pressure.
6. At 4 h, obtain samples for aldosterone levels and BMP.

Patient label: _____

Orders: _____

Ordering Provider's Signature: _____ Date: _____

Saline suppression	Baseline	4 h
Aldosterone		
Potassium		
Blood pressure		

References

1. Funder JW, Carey RM, Fardella C, et al. Case detection, diagnosis, and treatment of patients with primary aldosteronism: An endocrine society clinical practice guideline. J Clin Endocrinol Metab. 2008;93(9):3266–81.
2. Giacchetti G, Ronconi V, Lucarelli G, Boscaro M, Mantero F. Analysis of screening and confirmatory tests in the diagnosis of primary aldosteronism: need for a standardized protocol. J Hypertens. 2006;24(4):737–45.
3. Holland OB, Brown H, Von Kuhnert L, Fairchild C, Risk M, Gomez-Sanchez CE. Further evaluation of saline infusion for the diagnosis of primary aldosteronism. Hypertension. 1984;6(5) (Part 1):717–23.
4. McKenzie CA, Wright-Pascoe R, Boyne MS. Prospective evaluation and characteristics of patients with suspected primary hyperaldosteronism. West Indian Med J. 2007;56(3):258–63.

Chapter 16
Oral Sodium Loading Test

Indication: Confirmatory test for suspected primary aldosteronism (PA).

Materials Needed: Jug for 24 h urine collection.

> **Aldosterone:**
> Lavender top

Assay for Aldosterone: Enzymatic Radioimmunoassay (RIA).

Precautions: Do not perform this test in patients with severe uncontrolled hypertension, renal insufficiency, cardiac insufficiency, cardiac arrhythmia, or severe hypokalemia [1].

Interpretation: With concomitant urinary sodium excretion > 200 mEq/24 h and creatinine > 15 mg/kg/24 h for men and 10 mg/kg/24 h for women respectively; PA is unlikely if urinary aldosterone is <10 mcg/24 hr. Elevated urinary aldosterone excretion >12 mcg/24 h makes PA highly likely [1].

Caveats:

- This test is the most cost-effective test, but the conditions are not strictly controlled and patient compliance on urine collection is a potential limitation [2].
- Stop all potassium sparing and potassium wasting diuretics for 4 weeks. Stop beta-adrenergic blockers, central alpha-2 agonists (e.g., clonidine, alpha-methyldopa), non-steroidal anti-inflammatory drugs, angiotensin-converting enzyme inhibitors, angiotensin receptor blockers, renin inhibitors, dihydropyridine calcium channel antagonists for 2 weeks [1]. Blood pressure can be controlled with one or more of the following agents: verapamil extended release, selective alpha-1 blocker (e.g. Doxazosin), and hydralazine [1].

© Springer International Publishing Switzerland 2015
A. B. Ergin et al., *The Cleveland Clinic Manual of Dynamic Endocrine Testing,*
DOI 10.1007/978-3-319-13048-4_16

- In the presence of renal disease urinary aldosterone levels may be falsely low [1].
- When aldosterone levels are indeterminate (urinary aldosterone excretion 10–12 mcg/24 h) other confirmatory tests should be performed such as the IV saline loading test or the Captopril challenge test [1]. Although the Fludrocortisone suppression test may have a better diagnostic accuracy, it requires hospitalization and is generally not performed in North America.

Procedure [1]:

1. Patients should increase their sodium intake to >200 mmol (~6 g) per day for 3 days. Hint: 1 flat teaspoon equals 2.3 g of salt. In circumstances of high sodium dietary intolerance, patients can be given oral sodium chloride tablets (two 1 g sodium chloride tablets taken three times daily with food)
2. A basic metabolic panel (BMP) should be obtained prior to the start of the test to make sure that serum potassium is normal.
3. Patients should receive adequate slow-release potassium chloride supplementation to maintain plasma potassium in the normal range. Most patients may continue potassium intake during the salt loading.
4. Urinary aldosterone, sodium, potassium, and creatinine is measured in the 24 h urine collection from the morning of day 3 to the morning of day 4 and the jug is to be returned to the lab soon after collection is complete. Refrigerate urine during collection.
5. In patients with severe uncontrolled hypertension (BP>180/100 mmHg), delaying the test till better BP control is achieved, or proceeding with the Captopril challenge test may be considered.

Patient label: _____

Ordering Provider's Signature:_____Date:_____

Oral salt loading	Aldosterone	Potassium	Sodium
24 h urine			

References

1. Funder JW, Carey RM, Fardella C, et al. Case detection, diagnosis, and treatment of patients with primary aldosteronism: an endocrine society clinical practice guideline. J Clin Endocrinol Metab. 2008;93(9):3266–81.
2. Mulatero P, Monticone S, Bertello C, et al. Confirmatory tests in the diagnosis of primary aldosteronism. Horm Metab Res. 2010;42(6):406–10.

Chapter 17
Captopril Challenge Test

Indication:	Confirmation test for suspected aldosterone excess.
Preparation:	Patient should be sitting for an hour prior to the test.
Materials Needed:	Heplock/syringes/needle.

> **PRA and plasma aldosterone** can be sent in the same tube: **Lavender top** tube Transport: frozen (critical) Note: separate plasma from cells within 60 min of collection.

50 mg of captopril.

Blood tubes for plasma renin activity (PRA) and aldosterone.

Assay for PRA and Aldosterone:	Radioimmunoassay.
Precautions:	Monitor BP hourly.
Interpretation:	Plasma aldosterone is normally suppressed by captopril ($>30\%$). In patients with PA, aldosterone remains elevated (less than 30% suppression) and PRA remains suppressed [1–3]. In diagnosing APA, Post captopril A/R ratio >35 has sensitivity and specificity of 100% and 67.9% compared with 95.4% and 28.3% at baseline A/R ratio [3].

Caveats:

- There are reports of a substantial number of false negative or equivocal results [4, 5].

© Springer International Publishing Switzerland 2015
A. B. Ergin et al., *The Cleveland Clinic Manual of Dynamic Endocrine Testing*,
DOI 10.1007/978-3-319-13048-4_17

- In our institution we use this test when saline suppression or oral salt loading is not feasible or contraindicated such as in patients with uncontrolled blood pressure above 180/100.
- At low Na intake (<3 g/day), the saline suppression test (SST) has a higher negative predictive value than the Captopril challenge test. At a high sodium intake, SST offers no advantage over the easier-to-perform Captopril challenge test for the diagnosis of APA [3].
- Stop all potassium sparing diuretics for at least 4 weeks and stop potassium wasting diuretics, beta blockers, beta-adrenergic blockers, central alpha-2 agonists (e.g., clonidine, alpha-methyldopa), non-steroidal anti-inflammatory drugs, angiotensin-converting enzyme inhibitors, angiotensin receptor blockers, renin inhibitors, and dihydropyridine calcium channel antagonists for at least 2 weeks. Blood pressure can be controlled with verapamil, selective alpha 1 antagonists (e.g. prazosin, doxazosin, terazosin) or hydralazine in the meantime. Potassium levels should be corrected prior to the test [6].
- In patients with severe hypokalemia, a small dose of amiloride (≤5 mg) may be used to control hypokalemia while the patient undergoes confirmatory testing.

Procedure: Completed as outpatient.

1. Patient stays seated for 1 h prior to the initiation of the test.
2. Inset heplock and flush with 3–10 ml of normal saline as necessary.
3. Administer 50 mg captopril orally at time zero after drawing baseline blood samples for PRA and Aldosterone.
4. Draw blood for PRA and aldosterone at the 60th and 120th min.
5. Monitor BP and heart rate hourly.
6. Document the dose and time of captopril given and document the lab results and timing of results.
7. Discontinue heplock and discharge the patient

Patient label: _____

Documentation for medication orders:

Ordering provider's signature: _____Date: _____

Test results	Baseline	60 min	120 min
PRA			
Aldosterone			

References

1. Agharazii M, Douville P, Grose JH, Lebel M. Captopril suppression versus salt loading in confirming primary aldosteronism. Hypertension. 2001;37(6):1440–3.
2. Rossi E, Regolisti G, Negro A, Sani C, Davoli S, Perazzoli F. High prevalence of primary aldosteronism using postcaptopril plasma aldosterone to renin ratio as a screening test among italianhypertensives. Am J Hypertens. 2002;15(10):896–902.
3. Rossi GP, Belfiore A, Bernini G, et al. Comparison of the captopril and the saline infusion test for excluding aldosterone-producing adenoma. Hypertension. 2007;50(2):424–31.
4. Hambling C, Jung R, Gunn A, Browning M, Bartlett W. Re-evaluation of the captopril test for the diagnosis of primary hyperaldosteronism. Clin Endocrinol (Oxf). 1992;36(5):499–503.
5. Mulatero P, Bertello C, Garrone C, et al. Captopril test can give misleading results in patients with suspect primary aldosteronism. Hypertension. 2007;50(2):e26–7.
6. Funder JW, Carey RM, Fardella C, et al. Case detection, diagnosis, and treatment of patients with primary aldosteronism: an endocrine society clinical practice guideline. J Clin Endocrinol Metab. 2008;93(9):3266–81.

Chapter 18
Water Deprivation Test

Indication:
1. To confirm diagnosis of diabetes insipidus (DI).
2. To differentiate between central DI, nephrogenic DI, and primary polydipsia.

Patient Preparation: Initiation of the deprivation period depends on the severity of the DI; in routine cases, the patient may be made NPO after dinner or midnight. If polyuria is severe, start NPO early in the morning of the test (e.g., 6 am) [1]. Desmopressin must be stopped for at least 24 h prior to the test. Patients should also avoid alcohol, tobacco, and caffeine starting from the night prior to the test.

Materials Needed:

| Sodium: |
| gold top tube |
| Osmolality: |
| gold top tube |

1. Labels and requisitions *all marked STAT*.
2. Several serum separator tubes (SST) for sodium, labeled baseline and hourly.
3. Several SSTs for osmolality, labeled baseline and hourly.
4. Several urine cups for osmolality, labeled baseline and hourly.
5. Several plasma tubes for AVP.
6. DDAVP 2 mcg.
7. 500 cc 3 % saline, IV infusion set.
8. Heplock/syringes/needles.

Precautions: Severe dehydration (hypotension, tachycardia) may occur in patients with true diabetes insipidus. Weight loss should not be allowed to exceed 5 % of initial body weight and blood pressure should be monitored closely. Do not perform the water deprivation test in patients with renal insufficiency, uncontrolled diabetes mellitus, hypovolemia of any cause, untreated adrenal insufficiency, and hypothyroidism.

© Springer International Publishing Switzerland 2015   71
A. B. Ergin et al., *The Cleveland Clinic Manual of Dynamic Endocrine Testing,*
DOI 10.1007/978-3-319-13048-4_18

Interpretation: Normal response: Urine osmolality >600 mOsm/kg.

1. If serum osmolality goes above 300 mOsm/kg or serum sodium goes above (upper limit of normal) ULN while urine osmolality is less than 300 mOsm/kg **primary polydipsia, partial neurogenic**, and **partial nephrogenic** DI *are excluded*, and a challenge test with dDAVP 2 mcg SC is required.

   • DDAVP response, 2 h after DDAVP administration: higher than 50% increase in urine osmolality indicates **central DI (CDI)** and less than 10% increase strongly suggests **complete nephrogenic DI (NDI)** [1, 2].

2. If urine osmolality rises above 300 mOsm/kg before serum sodium is above the upper limit of normal; **complete neurogenic** and **complete nephrogenic DI are excluded**. Start 3% saline infusion or extend the test if 3% saline infusion is not possible. Once serum sodium or osmolality goal is achieved, draw blood for plasma AVP level and serum osmolality, and then administer DDAVP to see the response to DDAVP. See Figs. 18.1 and 18.2.

Caveats:

1. *In most patients, differentiation between different etiologies of DI may be reached by careful review of medical history and prior work up without a need for performing water deprivation test.*
2. If basal serum sodium concentration is above normal while the urine osmolality is below 300 mOsm/kg H2O, this test is unnecessary and can be potentially harmful. In this case, skip to the dDAVP challenge test.
3. Observation of the patient for the entire duration of the test is needed to prevent surreptitious drinking and non-osmotic stimulants of AVP secretion such as smoking, postural hypotension, vaso-vagal reactions, nausea, and hypotension.
4. If an episode of hypotension or nausea occurs, the entire test may be invalid, and it may need to be repeated on another day.
5. Complete emptying of the bladder during each collection should be ensured because the residual volume left in the bladder may dilute the urine of the next collection, and affect test interpretation. If incomplete emptying is suspected, creatinine concentration should be measured on each urine sample. Urine creatinine concentration multiplied by the urine volume should be quite constant.
6. Plasma AVP should be measured from heparinized blood. Plasma levels from samples processed with EDTA should not be used because they may contain variable artifacts that raise osmolality.
7. The osmometer for measurement of serum osmolality needs to be calibrated frequently against standard solutions. However, most hospital laboratories are unable to provide this degree of precision. Therefore it is better to rely on measurements of serum sodium concentration, which are determined with sufficient accuracy by most routine hospital laboratories

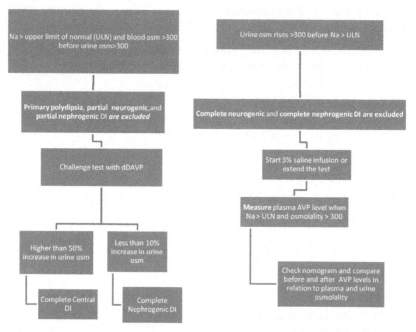

Fig. 18.1 Diagnostic algorithm for diabetes insipidus during water deprivation test

Water Deprivation Test in Patients with Diabetes Insipidus

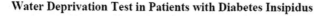

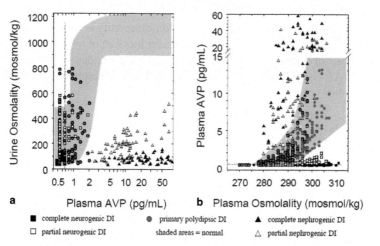

Fig. 18.2 Results of the water deprivation test on normal subjects (*shaded areas*) and patients with the three major forms of diabetes insipidus. Each plotted symbol represents a simultaneous sampling for two variables: plasma AVP (the antidiuretic hormone, arginine vasopressin) and urine osmolality (Fig. 18.1a), and plasma osmolality and plasma AVP (Fig. 18.1b). The *interrupted lines* denote the limit of the assay for plasma AVP; below the limiting value, no AVP can be detected in the plasma. (The data come from patients seen by Dr. Gary L. Robertson) [3]

Water Deprivation Test Procedure Start the test early in the morning. Observe the patient during the ENTIRE test. Do NOT leave the room unattended.

1. Record body weight and blood pressure after patient empties the bladder.
2. Calculate and document 95% of this weight on the patient's chart.
3. At baseline,

    a. Draw basic metabolic panel.
    b. Draw blood sample for STAT serum osmolality and sodium.
    c. Freeze 2 ml of plasma for later assay of AVP.

4. Every 1 h:

    a. Record urine volume.
    b. Check urine osmolality STAT

5. Every 2 h:

    a. Record body weight and blood pressure.
    b. Check serum sodium and osmolality STAT.
    c. Freeze 2 ml of plasma for later assay of AVP.

6. Stop the test when:

    • The serum sodium is > ULN or
    • Body weight decreases by 5% or
    • The patient develops hypotension, SBP > 100.

7. Obtain a plasma AVP level at the end of the test when serum sodium is > ULN.
8. Administer dDAVP (2 μg) sc and continue following urine osmolality and volume every 30 min for an additional 2 h. At this point, the test is completed.

If the serum sodium stays < ULN or the serum osmolality is < 300 mOsm/kg H2O when the urine osmolality is > 300, then consider infusion of hypertonic saline (3% NaCl at a rate of 0.1 ml/kg/min for 1–2 h) to reach these endpoints. Measure serum sodium STAT every 30 min until Na+ is above ULN. Measure plasma AVP in the same samples.

Patient label: _____

Orders:

Ordering Provider's Signature: _____ Date: _____

Time	BP	Weight	Urine volume	Urine osmo-lality	Serum sodium	Serum osmo-lality	Plasma AVP basal	Plasma AVP post
Baseline								

95 % of initial body weight = _____

References

1. Verbalis JG. Management of disorders of water metabolism in patients with pituitary tumors. Pituitary. 2002;5(2):119–32.
2. Zerbe RL, Robertson GL. A comparison of plasma vasopressin measurements with a standard indirect test in the differential diagnosis of polyuria. N Engl J Med. 1981;305(26):1539–46.
3. Robertson GL, Valtin H. Water deprivation protocol. www.nccpeds.com/kidney/articles/water_deprivation_protocol_pdf (Approved by the Scientific Advisory Committee of the Diabetes Insipidus Foundation, Inc.).

Part II
Dynamic Tests in Thyroid Disorders

Chapter 19
Thyroid Cancer Follow-Up: Withdrawal Protocol

Day	Date	What to Do
0	Day and Date	Have baseline TSH and Thyroglobulin drawn if not done in the past 60 days. Stop L-thyroxine medication beginning on day 0
7	Day and Date	One week after stopping L-thyroxine, begin Cytomel 25 or 37.5 mcg per day (Circle one dose) for 2 weeks
21	Day and Date	Stop Cytomel
28	Day and Date	Start low Iodine diet
35	Day and Date	Have TSH, Thyroglobulin lab work
37	Day and Date	Start collecting (24 h urine for iodine/creatinine) from 8 A.M. to 8 A.M. (next day) take it to lab prior to appointment
38	Day and Date	Report to nuclear medicine for tracer dose of ^{131}I in preparation for neck scan next day
40	Day and Date	Report to nuclear medicine for a whole body scan in the morning (48 h after tracer dose ingestion). You may receive RAI treatment dose on this day, if indicated as per your endocrinologis. If female age is <55, have pregnancy test done prior
	Day and Date	Report to nuclear medicine for total body scan if you have received radioactive iodine treatment dose

Start LOW IODINE DIET Date: _____

Name and Signature, RN: _____

Name and Signature, MD: _____

© Springer International Publishing Switzerland 2015

A. B. Ergin et al., *The Cleveland Clinic Manual of Dynamic Endocrine Testing*,
DOI 10.1007/978-3-319-13048-4_19

Chapter 20
Thyroid Cancer Follow-Up: Thyrogen Injection with No Scan

Day	Date	What to do
1	Day and date	Have labs (thyroglobulin) drawn
		If female of age 55 or under, have a pregnancy test done prior to thyrogen injection
		First thyrogen injection given by the nurse
2	Day and date	Second thyrogen injection given by the nurse
5	Day and date	Have labs (thyroglobulin) drawn at main campus or satellite

Name and Signature, RN: _____

Name and Signature, MD: _____

© Springer International Publishing Switzerland 2015
A. B. Ergin et al., *The Cleveland Clinic Manual of Dynamic Endocrine Testing,*
DOI 10.1007/978-3-319-13048-4_20

Chapter 21
Thyroid Cancer Follow-Up: Thyrogen Injection with Scan With/Without Treatment

Day	Date and time	What to do
−14	Day and date	Start with low-iodine diet. Continue this diet until after you have your blood work done on Day 5
1	Day and date	Have labs (TSH and thyroglobulin) drawn in the morning prior to thyrogen injection
		If female of age 55 or under, have a pregnancy test done prior to thyrogen injection
		First thyrogen injection given by nurse in the morning. Come back tomorrow for the second thyrogen injection
2	Day and date	Second thyrogen injection given by nurse in the morning
		Report to nuclear medicine for a radioactive iodine (RAI) tracer dose in the afternoon
3	Day and date	Report to nuclear edicine for a whole body scan in the morning (48 h after tracer dose ingestion). You may receive RAI treatment dose on this day, if indicated as per your endocrinologist. If female age is < 55, have a pregnancy test done prior
5	Day and date	Have labs (thyroglobulin) drawn 72 h after you had your injections
		You may stop your low-iodine diet after your blood work

Name and Signature, RN: _____

Name and Signature, MD: _____

© Springer International Publishing Switzerland 2015
A. B. Ergin et al., *The Cleveland Clinic Manual of Dynamic Endocrine Testing*,
DOI 10.1007/978-3-319-13048-4_21

Reconstitution, Preparation, and Administration of THYROGEN (Obtained from Prescribing Information)

The supplied lyophilized powder must be reconstituted with sterile water for injection. THYROGEN should be prepared and administered in the following manner:

- Add 1.2 mL of sterile water for injection to the vial containing the THYROGEN-lyophilized powder.
- Swirl the contents of the vial until all materials are dissolved. Do not shake the solution. The reconstituted THYROGEN solution has a concentration of 0.9 mg of thyrotropin alfa per mL.
- Visually inspect the reconstituted solution for a particulate matter and discoloration prior to administration. The reconstituted THYROGEN solution should be clear and colorless. Do not use if the solution has a particulate matter or is cloudy or discolored.
- Withdraw 1 mL of the reconstituted THYROGEN solution (0.9 mg of thyrotropin alfa) and inject intramuscularly in the buttocks. The reconstituted THYROGEN solution must be injected within 3 h unless refrigerated; if refrigerated, the reconstituted solution may be kept for up to 24 h.
- Discard unused portions. Do not mix with other substances.

Chapter 22
Levothyroxine Absorption Test

Indication:	To assess poor oral absorption of levothyroxine (LT4), and assist the clinician in differentiating true malabsorption from pseudomalabsorption (patient nonadherence).
Preparation:	Ten-hour fasting.
Materials Needed:	Hep-lock/syringes/needle

Total T4:
Electro
chemilumi-
nescence
Imunoassay,
light green
top.
Transport:
refrigerated

1000 mcg of LT4

Blood tubes for total or freeT4 measurement

Precautions:	Supervise patient continuously during the procedure.
Interpretation:	Absorption is calculated by using the following formula [1]:

$$\% LT4 \text{ absorption} = [(\text{peak}\Delta \text{ Total or free T4} \times \text{vd (dL)} \div \text{administered dose of LT4 } (\mu g)] \times 100].$$

Volume of distribution (Vd) in deciliters: $4.42 \times$ body mass index [1].

More than 60–80 % absorption is considered normal and rules out levothyroxine malabsorption [2, 3].

© Springer International Publishing Switzerland 2015
A. B. Ergin et al., *The Cleveland Clinic Manual of Dynamic Endocrine Testing*,
DOI 10.1007/978-3-319-13048-4_22

Biological Causes of Levothyroxine Malabsorption or change in metabolism or requirement [4]

Gastrointestinal Diseases

Celiac disease

Lactose intolerance

Vitamin B12 deficiency

Intestinal infections

(Giardia lamblia)

Liver diseases such as cirrhosis

Obstructive liver disease

Pancreatic diseases—Pancreatic insufficiency

Previous gastrointestinal surgery jejunostomy

Jejunoileal bypass

Short bowel syndrome

Medication Interference

Cholestyramine

Colestipol

Aluminum hydroxide-containing antacids

Ferrous sulphate

Sucralphate

Propranolol

Laxatives

Calcium supplements

Lovastatin

Bile acid sequestrants [1].

Activated charcoal

Anion exchange resins

Phenytoin

Phenobarbital

Carbamazepine

Rifampin

Amiodarone

Estrogen therapy

Dietary Interference

Walnuts

Soybean

Prunes

Herbal remedies

Others

Congestive heart failure

Pregnancy

Caveats:

- Before proceeding with this test, the biological causes of levothyroxine malabsorption should be evaluated as listed below.
- Obesity may cause overestimation of absorption.
- This test is not a well-established test in clinical practice. The value of this test should be weighed against risks and cost in each individual patient.

Procedure:

1. Perform the test after an overnight fast.
2. Hold all nonessential medications.
3. Insert hep-lock and flush with 3–10 ml of normal saline as necessary.
4. Have patient ingest 1000 mcg of levothyroxine.
5. Draw blood for total T4 levels at baseline before ingestion of LT4.
6. Draw blood for total T4 levels hourly for 5 h.
7. Monitor BP and heart rate hourly.
8. Document the dose and time of LT4 given and also document the lab results with timings.
9. Discontinue hep-lock.

Patient label:_____

Documentation for medication orders:

Ordering provider's signature _____Date:_____

Dose, time and date of LT4 given- Dose: Time: Date:

Results	Baseline Time	60 min	120 min	180 min	240 min	300 min
TT4						

References

1. Singh N, Weisler SL, Hershman JM. The acute effect of calcium carbonate on the intestinal absorption of levothyroxine. Thyroid. 2001;11(10):967–71.
2. Fish LH, Schwartz HL, Cavanaugh J, Steffes MW, Bantle JP, Oppenheimer JH. Replacement dose, metabolism, and bioavailability of levothyroxine in the treatment of hypothyroidism. N Engl J Med. 1987;316(13):764–70.
3. Wenzel KW, Kirschsieper HE. Aspects of the absorption of oral L-thyroxine in normal man. Metab Clin Exp. 1977;26(1):1–8.
4. Lips D, Van Reisen M, Voigt V, Venekamp W. Diagnosis and treatment of levothyroxine pseudomalabsorption. Neth J Med. 2004;62(4):114–8.

Part III
Dynamic Tests in Glucose Metabolism/ Pancreas Disorders

Chapter 23
Seventy Two Hours Fast for Insulinoma

Indication:	To confirm and determine the cause of suspected spontaneous hypoglycemia.
Contraindication:	Pregnancy, liver or kidney failure, unstable angina.
Preparation:	No special preparation is needed. Patient can have breakfast on the day of testing if hypoglycemia develops frequently.
Materials Needed:	Blood tubes in sufficient amount for testing should be ready at bedside:

Maximum of three tubes to be used for one set of testing: one gold top tube for insulin, pro-insulin, and c-peptide in addition to a grey top tube for fasting blood glucose (BG), green top tube for beta-hydroxybutyrate.

Insulin: Gold top tube, 1 ml. Methodology: chemiluminescence immunoassay

Pro-insulin gold top tube, 1 ml. Assay: methodology: chemiluminescence immunoassay transport: centrifuge, aliquot, and freeze (keep in ice until delivered to the lab)

C-Peptide: Gold top tube, 1 ml. Methodology: chemiluminescence immunoassay

Fasting glucose grey-top tube, 1 ml. Methodology: glucose hexokinase

Beta hydroxybutyrate green-top tube, 1 ml. Methodology: enzymatic

A syringe containing 50% glucose solution.

Glucagon 1 mg intravenously injectable.

Heplock/syringes/needle

© Springer International Publishing Switzerland 2015
A. B. Ergin et al., *The Cleveland Clinic Manual of Dynamic Endocrine Testing*,
DOI 10.1007/978-3-319-13048-4_23

Precautions: All patients must be warned that they will be fasting, and
                              unable to leave the clinic/ward unaccompanied during the
                              test before starting.

                              Have D50 and glucagon ampule ready in case of emergency.

Interpretation: See table [1] below for interpretation.

Symptoms, signs, or both	Glucose (mg/dl)	Insulin (μU/ml)	C-peptide (nmol/liter)	Proinsulin (pmol/liter)	β-Hydroxy-butyrate (mmol/liter)	Glucose increase after glucagon (mg/dl)	Circulating oral hypo-glycemic	Antibody to insulin	Diagnostic inter-pretation
No	< 55	< 3	< 0.2	< 5	> 2.7	< 25	No	No	Normal
Yes	< 55	» 3	< 0.2	< 5	≤ 2.7	> 25	No	Neg (Pos)	Exogenous insulin
Yes	< 55	≥ 3	≥ 0.2	≥ 5	≤ 2.7	> 25	No	Neg	Insulinoma, NIPHS, PGBH
Yes	< 55	≥ 3	≥ 0.2	≥ 5	≤ 2.7	> 25	Yes	Neg	Oral hypo-glycemic agent
Yes	< 55	» 3	» 0.2^a	» 5^a	≤ 2.7	> 25	No	Pos	Insulin autoimmune
Yes	< 55	< 3	< 0.2	< 5	≤ 2.7	> 25	No	Neg	IGF^b
Yes	< 55	< 3	< 0.2	< 5	> 2.7	< 25	No	Neg	Not insulin (or IGF)-mediated

Neg, negative; Pos, positive; PGBH, post gastric bypass hypoglycemia.
a Free C-peptide and proinsulin concentrations are low.
b Increased pro-IGF-II, free IGF-II, IGF-II/IGF-I ratio.

Caveats:

- It is equally important that the blood samples and laboratory slips be carefully
  labeled, particularly with the exact time, and that the labeling information be
  recorded on a flow sheet. Later interpretation of the results is possible only with
  this detail.
- Young, lean, healthy women may have plasma glucose concentrations in the
  range of 40 mg/dL (2.2 mmol/L) or even lower after prolonged periods of fasting
  [2]. A low plasma glucose value is necessary but not sufficient for the diagnosis
  of hypoglycemia. ***Do not stop the tests other than the conditions specified in
  the procedure.*** Careful questioning and testing for subtle symptoms or signs
  of hypoglycemia should be conducted repeatedly when the patient's plasma
  glucose is near or in the hypoglycemic range.
- The sensitivity and specificity of the established diagnostic parameters: Insulin
  (≥3 μU/ml), 93 and 95%; C-peptide (≥0.2 nmol/ml), 100 and 60%; proinsulin
  (≥5 pmol/L), 100 and 68%; BHOB (≤2.7 mmol/L), 100 and 100%; and plasma
  glucose response to iv glucagon (≥25 mg/dl), 91 and 95%, respectively [3].
- The specificity of these parameters was improved when compared with normal
  patients whose plasma glucose at the end of a prolonged fast was 50 mg/dl or

less: insulin, 100 %; C-peptide, 78 %; proinsulin, 78 %; and glucose response to glucagon, 100 % [3].

- About 6 % of insulinomas present as postprandial hypoglycemia, and other disorders such as nesidioblastosis may also present with postprandial hypoglycemia. Mixed meal test may have a role in evaluation of such patients.

Procedure:

1. Date the last ingestion of calories.

2. Document the baseline vital signs.

3. Stop all foods and drinks except calorie free and caffeine free beverages and water.

4. Ensure that the patient is active during waking hours.

5. Insert heplock.

6. Flush heplock with 3–10 cc ml normal saline as needed.

7. Draw blood for baseline labs for *5 tests*: **insulin, pro-insulin, C-peptide, fasting glucose, beta hydroxybutyrate.**

8. Check finger stick blood sugar every 2 h until BG is 60 mg/dl or less.

9. Check finger stick blood sugar every 1 h after BG is 60 mg/dl or less.

10. Send stat blood for the *5 tests* as above after fingerstick BG is less than 60 mg/dl and then every 1 h (insulin, glucose, c-peptide, beta hydroxy butyrate). *Samples should be analyzed only in those samples in which the plasma glucose concentration is less than 45 mg/dl (2.5 mmol/L).*

    Important note: The decision to end the fast must not be made on the basis of a fingerstick BG value. If it is judged necessary to treat urgently because of severe symptoms, obtain samples for all the tests noted above before administering carbohydrates.

    Recommend to draw blood twice a day regardless of BG levels. In some cases the trend in the levels can help clinicians with interpretation,

11. End the fasting when:

    • plasma glucose concentration is ≤45 mg/dL (2.5 mmol/L) in plasma (not in fingestick) *in an asymtopmatic patient after careful evaluation (see caveats)* or
    • patient has symptoms or signs of hypoglycemia when BG is ≤45 mg/dL in plasma or
    • plasma glucose concentration is less than 55 mg/dL (3 mmol/L) if Whipple's triad was documented on a prior occasion or
    • 72 h have elapsed

After ending the test send blood samples STAT for the following:

Insulin, pro-insulin, C-peptide, fasting glucose, beta hydroxybutyrate, and hypoglycemia panel that include sulfonylurea screen and other insulin secretagogues.

12. Give 1 mg glucagon intravenously and recheck plasma glucose 10, 20, and 30 min later. Patient should be then fed right away after last blood draw.

Patient label: _____

Documentation for medication orders: _____

Ordering Provider's Signature: _____ Date: _____

Glucose (Time) e.g 45 (3:12	Symptoms Y/N	Insulin	C-peptide	Proinsulin	B-OH butyrate	BG increase after glucagon > 25mg/dl Y/N	Antibody to insulin Y/N	SU screen positive Y/N

References

1. Cryer PE, Axelrod L, Grossman AB, Heller SR, Montori VM, Seaquist ER. Evaluation and management of adult hypoglycemic disorders: an endocrine society clinical practice guideline. J Clin Endocrinol Metab. 2009;94(3):709–28.
2. Merimee TJ, Fineberg SE. Homeostasis during fasting. II. Hormone substrate differences between men and women. J Clin Endocrinol Metab. 1973;37(5):698–702.
3. Placzkowski KA, Vella A, Thompson GB, et al. Secular trends in the presentation and management of functioning insulinoma at the mayo clinic, 1987–2007. J Clin Endocrinol Metab. 2009;94(4):1069–73.

Chapter 24
Glucagon Stimulation

Indication:	Assessment of beta cell reserve.
Contraindication:	Patients with type 1 diabetes mellitus.
Preparation [1:]	NPO except water after midnight and during the test.
	Ten hours after the last dose of short-acting or intermediate-acting insulin, metformin or thiazolidinedione.
	At least 24 h after a dose of sulfonylurea or long-acting insulin (glargine or detemir).
Materials Needed:	Three gold top tubes, glucagon
	C-peptide: Gold top tube
	Transport: Refrigerated.
Assay for C-peptide:	Chemiluminescence immunoassay.
Precautions:	None.
Interpretation:	Beta Cell functional reserve was defined as preserved if the peak C-peptide response to glucagon is at least 1.5 ng/dL (0.5 nmol/L) or fasting C-peptide concentration of at least 1 ng/dL (0.33 nmol/L). Beta cell functional reserve is defined as absent if the glucagon stimulated or fasting C-peptide concentrations do not meet these criteria [1].
	Patients who do not have preserved beta cell function by the above protocol should not undergo a trial of insulin withdrawal.

© Springer International Publishing Switzerland 2015
A. B. Ergin et al., *The Cleveland Clinic Manual of Dynamic Endocrine Testing*,
DOI 10.1007/978-3-319-13048-4_24

Caveats:

- Above cut-points were established using the radioimmunoassay (RIA) for human C-peptide. They have been shown to accurately predict beta cell function and glycemic control after 1 year [2, 3]; however, they have not as yet been standardized across other newer C-peptide immuunoassays.
- Measurement of beta cell antibodies also helps in understanding underlying pathology although immediate insulin dependence can be more sharply estimated by measurement of basal or stimulated C-peptide levels.
- For patients with diabetic ketoacidosis (DKA) and the typical type 1 diabetes clinical phenotype (young, thin), it may not be necessary to measure C-peptide levels. These patients should be maintained on insulin.

Procedure:

1. Ensure patient is fasting from midnight.
2. Weigh patient and document it.
3. Insert intravenous cannula (hep-lock) for intravenous access between 7:30–8 A.M.
4. Obtain baseline C-peptide levels.
5. Administer glucagon intravenously 1 mg. Confirm the medication doses with physician.
6. Obtain blood samples for C-peptide 5 and 10 min after the glucagon infusion.
7. Discontinue hep-lock.

Patient label: _____

Documentation for medication orders: _____

Ordering provider's signature: _____ Date: _____

Glucagon stim test	Time	C-peptide
Basal (0 min)		
5 min		
10 min		

References

1. Maldonado M, Hampe CS, Gaur LK, et al. Ketosis-prone diabetes: dissection of a heterogeneous syndrome using an immunogenetic and β-cell functional classification, prospective analysis, and clinical outcomes. J Clin Endocrinol Metab. 2003;88(11):5090–8.
2. Balasubramanyam A, Garza G, Rodriguez L, et al. Accuracy and predictive value of classification schemes for ketosis-prone diabetes. Diabetes Care. 2006;29(12):2575–9.
3. Maldonado M, D'Amico S, Otiniano M, Balasubramanyam A, Rodriguez L, Cuevas E. Predictors of glycaemic control in indigent patients presenting with diabetic ketoacidosis. Diabetes Obes Metab. 2005;7(3):282–9.

Chapter 25
Mixed Meal Hypoglycemia Test

Indication:	Patients with suspected postprandial hypoglycemia.
Preparation:	10 h fasting.
Materials needed:	Ensure plus high protein drink (6 ml/kg with max dose of 360 ml)
	Blood tubes in sufficient amount for testing should be ready at bedside:
	Maximum three tubes for one set of testing: One gold top tube for insulin, pro-insulin and c-peptide, grey top tube for fasting BG, and green top tube for beta-hydroxybutyrate.
	Insulin: gold top tube, methodology: chemiluminescence immunoassay
	Pro-insulin gold top tube, methodology: Chemiluminescence immunoassay, transport: centrifuge, aliquot and freeze (keep on ice until delivered to the lab)
	C-Peptide: gold top tube, methodology: chemiluminescence immunoassay
	Fasting glucose: grey top tube, Methodology Glucose hexokinase
	Beta hydroxybutyrate: green top tube. Methodology Enzymatic
	A syringe containing 50% glucose solution.
	Glucagon 1 mg intravenously injectable.
	Heplock/syringes/needle.
Precautions:	Have D50 and some fruit juice ready in case of emergency.
Interpretation:	Standards for the interpretation of the mixed-meal test have not been established. Current clinical usage is to apply the same criteria developed under fasting conditions for insulinoma to the results from a mixed-meal challenge [1]. See Table 1 for interpretation.

© Springer International Publishing Switzerland 2015
A. B. Ergin et al., *The Cleveland Clinic Manual of Dynamic Endocrine Testing,*
DOI 10.1007/978-3-319-13048-4_25

Table 1 Patterns of findings during fasting or after a mixed meal in normal individuals with no symptoms or signs despite relatively low plasma glucose concentrations (i.e., Whipple's triad not documented) and in individuals with hyperinsulinemic (or IGF-mediated) hypoglycemia or hypoglycemia caused by other mechanisms

Symptoms, signs, or both	Glucose (mg/dl)	Insulin (µU/ml)	C-peptide (nmol/liter)	Proinsulin (pmol/liter)	β-Hydroxy-butyrate (mmol/liter)	Glucose increase after glucagon (mg/dl)	Circulating oral hypo-glycemic	Antibody to insulin	Diagnostic inter-pretation
No	< 55	< 3	< 0.2	< 5	> 2.7	< 25	No	No	Normal
Yes	< 55	» 3	< 0.2	< 5	≤ 2.7	> 25	No	Neg (Pos)	Exogenous insulin
Yes	< 55	≥ 3	≥ 0.2	≥ 5	≤ 2.7	> 25	No	Neg	Insulinoma, NIPHS, PGBH
Yes	< 55	≥ 3	≥ 0.2	≥ 5	≤ 2.7	> 25	Yes	Neg	Oral hypo-glycemic agent
Yes	< 55	» 3	» 0.2^a	» 5^a	≤ 2.7	> 25	No	Pos	Insulin autoimmune
Yes	< 55	< 3	< 0.2	< 5	≤ 2.7	> 25	No	Neg	IGF^b
Yes	< 55	< 3	< 0.2	< 5	> 2.7	< 25	No	Neg	Not insulin (or IGF)-mediated

Neg, negative; Pos, positive; PGBH, post gastric bypass hypoglycemia.
a Free C-peptide and proinsulin concentrations are low.
b Increased pro-IGF-II, free IGF-II, IGF-II/IGF-I ratio.

If a patient is symptomatic and blood glucose is normal, diagnosis of postprandial syndrome can be made.

Caveats:

- An oral glucose tolerance test should never be used for the evaluation of suspected postprandial hypoglycemia [2] because the nadir for blood glucose concentration after the ingestion of 100 g of glucose may fall into the hypoglycemia range in normal, asymptomatic individuals [3].
- Postprandial (reactive) hypoglycemia is a descriptor of the timing of hypoglycemia and is not a diagnosis. When biochemical evidence of postprandial hypoglycemia is confirmed, the cause must be determined. Samples should be analyzed only in those time points in which the plasma glucose concentration is less than 45 mg/dl (2.5 m mol/l).

Procedure:

1. Perform the test after an overnight fast.
2. Hold all nonessential medications.
3. Have the patient drink ensure plus high protein drink (6 ml/kg with max dose of 360 ml).
4. Draw blood for plasma glucose, insulin, C-peptide, and proinsulin at 15, 30, 60, 90, and 120th minute and at 3rd, 4th, and finally at 5th hour (see number 7). Observe the patient for symptoms and/or signs of hypoglycemia, and ask the patient to keep a written log of all symptoms, timed from the start of meal ingestion. If possible, avoid providing carbohydrate or food until the test is completed [4].
5. If it is necessary to treat a patient because of severe symptoms prior to the end of the test, obtain samples for plasma glucose, insulin, C-peptide, and proinsulin before administering carbohydrates.
6. Samples for plasma insulin, C-peptide, and proinsulin should be sent for analysis only for those sampleswhich have plasma glucose less than 60 mg/dl (3.3 m mol/l).
7. Send blood for sulfonyluera and metiglinide panel.

Glucose(Time)	Symptoms	Insulin	C -peptide	Proinsulin	B -OH butyrate	BG increase after glucagon>25mg/dl Y/N	Antibody to insulin Y/N	SU screen positive Y/N
e.g 45(3:12 p)	Y/N							

Patient label:_____

RN performing the procedure:_____

Ordering Provider's Signature: _____Date:_____

References

1. Service F. Hypoglycemic disorders. N Engl J Med. 1995;332(17):1144–52.
2. Hogan MJ, Service FJ, Sharbrough FW, Gerich JE. Oral glucose tolerance test compared with a mixed meal in the diagnosis of reactive hypoglycemia. A caveat on stimulation. Mayo Clin Proc. 1983;58(8):491–6.
3. Lev-Ran A, Anderson RW. The diagnosis of postprandial hypoglycemia. Diabetes. 1981;30(12):996–9.
4. Cryer PE, Axelrod L, Grossman AB, Heller SR, Montori VM, Seaquist ER. Evaluation and management of adult hypoglycemic disorders: An endocrine society clinical practice guideline. J Clin Endocrinol Metab. 2009;94(3):709–28.

Chapter 26
Secretin Stimulation Test

Indication:	This test is performed in order to differentiate gastrinomas from other causes of hypergastrinemia.
Preparation:	NPO except water after midnight and during the test. Tapering patients off proton pump inhibitors (PPI) by replacing them with other antacids is preferable.
Materials Needed:	Seven gold top tubes, Secretin.
	Gastrin: Gold top tube. Transport: Frozen, separate serum from cell as soon as possible.
Assay for Gastrin:	Radioimmunoassay (RIA).
Precautions:	None.
Interpretation:	A rise in gastrin level > 120 pg/ml compared to baseline at any point of time post-secretin infusion has 94% sensitivity and 100% specificity to diagnose gastrinoma [1].

Caveats:

- The standard secretin stimulation test is performed with patients off antacids and anticholinergics for at least 12 h. Although some experts suggests that PPI does not interfere with interpretation of gastrin levels during secretin stimulation testing, others recommend gradual tapering of PPI to prevent a rebound increase in gastric acid secretion [2]. This area is not adequately studied.
- Serum chromogranin A levels, although nonspecific, may support a diagnosis of neuroendocrine tumor, especially if significant elevated [3].
- Gastrin levels usually peak in the first 2–10 min.

© Springer International Publishing Switzerland 2015
A. B. Ergin et al., *The Cleveland Clinic Manual of Dynamic Endocrine Testing*,
DOI 10.1007/978-3-319-13048-4_26

Procedure [1]:

1. Ensure that patient fasts from midnight.
2. Insert intravenous cannula (heplock) for intravenous access.
3. Obtain two baseline gastrin levels.
4. Administer secretin 0.4 µg/kg intravenously over 1 min. Confirm the medication doses with physician.
5. Obtain blood samples for gastrin 2, 5, 10, 15, and 20 min after the secretin infusion.
6. Discontinue heplock.

Patient label:_____

Documentation for medication orders:_____

Ordering Provider's Signature: _____Date:_____

Glucagon stim test	Time	Gastrin
Basal(0 min)-twice		
2 min		
5 min		
10 min		
15 min		
20 min		

References

1. McGuigan JE, Wolfe MM. Secretin injection test in the diagnosis of gastrinoma. Gastroenterology. 1980;79(6):1324–31.
2. Désir B, Poitras P. Oral pantoprazole for acid suppression in the treatment of patients with Zollinger-Ellison syndrome. Can J Gastroenterol. 2001;15(12):795–8.
3. Nobels FR, Kwekkeboom DJ, Coopmans W, Schoenmakers CH, Lindemans J, DeHerder WW, Krenning EP, Bouillon R, Lamberts SW. Chromogranin A as serum marker for neuroendocrine neoplasia: comparison with neuron-specific enolase and the alpha-subunit of glycoprotein hormones. J Clin Endocrinol Metab. 1997;82(8):2622–8.

Part IV
Invasive Dynamic Endocrine Testing

Chapter 27
Inferior Petrosal Sinus Sampling

Indication: In order to differentiate between ectopic ACTH syndrome (EAS) and Cushing's disease (CD) in patients with ACTH-dependent Cushing's syndrome.

Preparation: Patient should be in fasting state. The authors measure serum cortisol level in the morning of the day inferior petrosal sinus sampling (IPSS) is planned and only proceed with the procedure if cortisol is > 10 mcg/dL. Most patients have a cortisol > 15 mcg/dL.

Precautions: The incidence of serious complications, such as a cerebrovascular accident, is 0.2 % when the procedure is performed by an experienced radiologist [3].

Interpretation: A central-to-peripheral plasma ACTH gradient of ≥2.0 before CRH administration, or ≥3.0 after corticotropin-releasing hormone (CRH) establishes a pituitary source of ACTH; the gradient is usually much greater, especially after CRH injection.

© Springer International Publishing Switzerland 2015
A. B. Ergin et al., *The Cleveland Clinic Manual of Dynamic Endocrine Testing*,
DOI 10.1007/978-3-319-13048-4_27

Caveats:

- Sensitivity and specificity of IPSS is > 88% and close to 100% after CRH administration respectively [1].
- In cases where the IPS to peripheral (IPS:P) ACTH gradient is not consistent with a pituitary source, peripheral ACTH response (> 35%) to CRH administration suggests central etiology rather than ectopic source [5].
- Radiologic confirmation of placement of catheter tip in IPS may not be reliable [4].
- IPS:P prolactin ratios greater than 1.8, confirm accurate catheterization [2]. Most patients with appropriate IPS catheterization have a gradient > 1.3 [5]. Prolactin may be measured routinely during IPSS, or in order to cut back on the cost, be stored and measured later on if IPS:P ACTH ratio is not consistent with a pituitary source.
- In the absence of appropriate bilateral IPS catheterization, which may be confirmed by measurement of IPS:P prolactin ratio, a lack of significant IPS:P ACTH gradient does not rule a pituitary source as the underlying etiology for Cushing's syndrome. In addition, confirmation of accurate venous sampling in only one IPS may not rule out a pituitary source in the contralateral side of the pituitary gland due to variable venous drainage [4].
- Petrosal sinus sampling is of limited value in distinguishing between patients with Cushing's syndrome and normal individuals or those with pseudo-Cushing's states. Therefore, a diagnosis of ACTH-dependent Cushing's syndrome should be established before referring a patient for IPSS [6].

Procedure: An institution specific protocol should be developed by an interested group of endocrinologists, radiologists, and laboratory personnel.

Sample	ACTH (pg/mL)						Prolactin (ng/mL)					Cortisol (µg/mL)
	Peripheral	Petrosal sinus		ACTH ratio			Peripheral	Petrosal sinus		Prolactin ratio		Peripheral
		Right	Left	R/P	L/P	R/L		Right	Left	R/P	L/P	
ADH (−10 min)												
ADH (−5 min)												
ADH (+3 min)												
ADH (+5 min)												
ADH (+10 min)												

References

1. Colao A, Faggiano A, Pivonello R, et al. Inferior petrosal sinus sampling in the differential diagnosis of Cushing's syndrome: results of an Italian multicenter study. Eur J Endocrinol. 2001;144(5):499–507.
2. Findling JW, Kehoe ME, Raff H. Identification of patients with Cushing's disease with negative pituitary adrenocorticotropin gradients during inferior petrosal sinus sampling: prolactin as an index of pituitary venous effluent. J Clin Endocrinol Metab. 2004;89(12):6005–6009.
3. Miller DL, Doppman JL, Peterman SB, Nieman LK, Oldfield EH, Chang R. Neurologic complications of petrosal sinus sampling. Radiology. 1992;185(1):143–147.
4. Mulligan GB, Eray E, Faiman C, et al. Reduction of false-negative results in inferior petrosal sinus sampling with simultaneous prolactin and corticotropin measurement. Endocrine Practice. 2011;17(1):33–40.
5. Swearingen B, Katznelson L, Miller K, et al. Diagnostic errors after inferior petrosal sinus sampling. J Clin Endocrinol Metab. 2004;89(8):3752–3763.
6. Yanovski JA, Cutler GB, Jr, Doppman JL, et al. The limited ability of inferior petrosal sinus sampling with corticotropin-releasing hormone to distinguish Cushing's disease from pseudo-Cushing's states or normal physiology. J Clin Endocrinol Metab. 1993;77(2):503–509.

Chapter 28
Adrenal Venous Sampling

Indication: In order to distinguish between unilateral and bilateral adrenal disease in patients with primary aldosteronism [1].

Preparation: Patient should be in fasting state. The test should be done in the morning, with the patient in the supine position for at least 1 h before sampling [2]. Patient should be normokalemic prior to procedure.

Precautions: At centers with experience with AVS, the complication rate is 2.5% or less [3, 4].

Interpretation: 1. **Confirm successful catheterization**

With cosyntropin infusion, the adrenal vein (right and left) to IVC cortisol ratio is typically more than 10:1; a ratio of at least 3:1 is required to be confident that the adrenal veins were successfully catheterized [4]. When cosyntropin infusion is not used, an adrenal vein to IVC cortisol gradient of more than 2:1 is recommended [5, 6]. Most institutions perform AVS with cosyntropin stimulation.

2. **Correct aldosterone levels for cortisol and interpret A/C ratios in order to localize the tumor side.**

Dividing the right and left adrenal vein plasma aldosterone concentrations by same-sided cortisol concentrations (A/C ratio) corrects for the dilutional effect of the inferior phrenic vein flow into the left adrenal vein; these are termed cortisol-corrected ratios (A/C ratio).

When cosyntropin infusion used criteria for localization is a cut-off for the cortisol–corrected aldosterone ratio (A/C) from high side to low side of more than 4:1 to indicate unilateral aldosterone excess [2], the true positive rate is 88% [6].

© Springer International Publishing Switzerland 2015
A. B. Ergin et al., *The Cleveland Clinic Manual of Dynamic Endocrine Testing*,
DOI 10.1007/978-3-319-13048-4_28

- An A/C ratio less than 3.0 is consistent with bilateral aldosterone hypersecretion.
- Ratios between 3 and 4.0 represent a zone of overlap.

If the A/C ratio of low side is less than the IVC A/C ratio, the tumor will be on the contralateral site in 93 % of patients with surgically confirmed APA [4]. This criterion may be particularly helpful in patients with only unilateral successful adrenal vein catheterization.

Caveats:

- We do not recommend AVS testing without cosyntropin stimulation due to high false positive rates [7].
- Medications that may increase renin secretion (e.g., mineralocorticoid receptor (MR) antagonists [spironolactone and eplerenone], high-dose amiloride [i.e., > 5 mg/day], ACE inhibitors, ARBs, and renin inhibitors [e.g., aliskiren]) should be discontinued for at least 4 weeks before AVS until more data on the accuracy of AVS in their presence is available [2]. It is plausible that keeping a patient with a history of severe uncontrolled hypertension and/or hypokalemia on these agents may be allowed in the presence of low renin (< 1 ng/ml.hr) levels. However, wherever possible, MR antagonists should be avoided because they have the potential to allow a rise in renin secretion, which can stimulate aldosterone secretion from the unaffected side, thus minimizing the lateralization. Such an approach is in line with our institutional experience.
- Preferably, extended release verapamil, peripheral alpha adrenergic receptor antagonists (e.g. doxazosin, terazosin and prazosin), and hydralazine should be used for blood pressure control prior to AVS.

Procedure: An institution-specific protocol should be developed by an interested group of endocrinologists, radiologists, and laboratory personnel.

	Cortisol	Aldoste-rone	A/C	A/C dominant A/C non-dominant	A/C non dominant A/C AVC
Right AV					
Left AV					
Low IVC					

References

1. Funder JW, Carey RM, Fardella C, et al. Case detection, diagnosis, and treatment of patients with primary aldosteronism: an endocrine society clinical practice guideline. J Clin Endocrinol Metab. 2008;93(9):3266–81.
2. Young WF, Stanson AW. What are the keys to successful adrenal venous sampling (AVS) in patients with primary aldosteronism? Clin Endocrinol (Oxf). 2009;70(1):14–7.
3. Rossi GP, Pitter G, Bernante P, Motta R, Feltrin G, Miotto D. Adrenal vein sampling for primary aldosteronism: the assessment of selectivity and lateralization of aldosterone excess baseline and after adrenocorticotropic hormone (ACTH) stimulation. J Hypertens. 2008;26(5):989–97.
4. Young Jr WF, Stanson AW, Thompson GB, Grant CS, Farley DR, van Heerden JA. Role for adrenal venous sampling in primary aldosteronism. Surgery. 2004;136(6):1227–35.
5. Daunt N. Adrenal vein sampling: how to make it quick, easy, and successful. Radiographics. 2005;25 Suppl 1:S143–58.
6. Rossi et al. Hypertension. 2014;63:151–60.
7. Webb R, Mathur A, Chang R, et al. What is the best criterion for the interpretation of adrenal vein sample results in patients with primary hyperaldosteronism? Ann Surg Oncol. 2012;19(6):1881–6.

Index

© Springer International Publishing Switzerland 2015
A. B. Ergin et al., *The Cleveland Clinic Manual of Dynamic Endocrine Testing*,
DOI 10.1007/978-3-319-13048-4

Plasma glucose concentration 99
Plasma renin activity (PRA) 69
Postprandial (reactive) hypoglycemia 108

R
Radioimmunoassay (RIA) 11, 111

S
Saline suppression test (SST) 70

T
THYROGEN 86
Thyroid cancer follow-up 83, 85